MW01079389

see pg 584
RTP Bentel

An Atlas of
Brachytherapy

Basil S. Hilaris, M.D., FACR
Dattatreyudu Nori, M.D.
Lowell L. Anderson, Ph.D.

Memorial Sloan-Kettering Cancer Center

Cornell University Medical College
New York

Macmillan Publishing Company
New York
Collier Macmillan Canada, Inc.
Toronto
Collier Macmillan Publishers
London

Macmillan Publishing Company
866 Third Avenue, New York, New York 10022

Collier Macmillan Canada, Inc.
Collier Macmillan Publishers • London

Library of Congress Cataloging-in-Publication Data

Hilaris, Basil S., 1928–
    An atlas of brachytherapy/Basil S. Hilaris, Dattatreyudu Nori,
Lowell L. Anderson.
        p.   cm.
    Includes bibliographies and index.
    ISBN 0-02-354770-7
    1. Radioisotope brachytherapy—Atlases. 2. Cancer—Radiotherapy—
Atlases.   I. Nori, Dattatreyudu, 1947–   . II. Anderson, Lowell
L. III. Title.
    [DNLM: 1. Brachytherapy—atlases.   WN 17 H641a]
RC271.R27H54 1987
616.99′406424—dc19

Printing: 1 2 3 4 5 6 7 8   Year: 8 9 0 1 2 3 4 5 6

Contents

Introduction

"The various reasons we have just enumerated lead us to believe that the new radioactive substance contains a new element to which we propose to give the name of RADIUM" was announced by Marie and Pierre Curie at the meeting of the Academy of Science in Paris on December 26, 1898 (From: *Madame Curie*, by Eve Curie; published by Pocket Books, New York, 1967). It took another 45 months, however, before the Curies were able to prepare a tiny amount of pure radium and determine its atomic weight to be 226!! (**Fig. 1**, Left).

Following Becquerel's accidental radium burn, Pierre Curie, in 1901, deliberately produced a radium ulcer on his arm (Fig. 1, right). Shortly thereafter, in the same year, Pierre Curie gave a small radium tube to Dr. Danlos and suggested he insert it into a tumor.

THUS RADIUM THERAPY WAS BORN.

The early pioneers resorted to the method of inserting bulky radium tubes within the tumor for a certain period of time and then withdrew them.

In 1914, Stevenson and Joly improved the technique by using pure radium sulfate, thus manufacturing the first radium "needles" made of steel or platinum.

A different method was worked out during the same period at Memorial Hospital by Failla, who collected radon gas in tiny glass tubes that were then inserted into tumors and left there indefinitely. The Memorial Hospital experience with "radium needles" and "radon seeds" was reported in 1917 by Janeway, Barringer, and Failla (**Fig. 2**).

Initially, the number of milligrams employed and the duration of the treatment led to a dosage specification expressed in terms of "milligram, hours".

Early attempts to develop "biological" units of radium therapy, i.e., the amount of radiation necessary to eradicate a mouse cancer, were not practical.

Likewise, "physical" units, i.e., measurements with an ionization chamber or measurements of heat produced by the absorption of radiation, could not give useful results.

A practical approach was found by specifying the exposure in milligram-hours that would result in a skin reaction at a distance of 2 cm. Thus, the "erythema dose" was born.

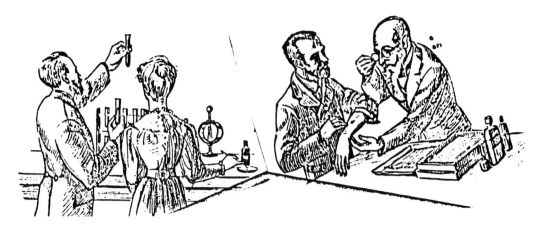

Discovery of radium by
P. and M. Curie (1898).

Following Becquerel's accidental
radium burn, Pierre Curie deliberately produced a radium ulcer on
his arm...(1901).

FIGURE 1

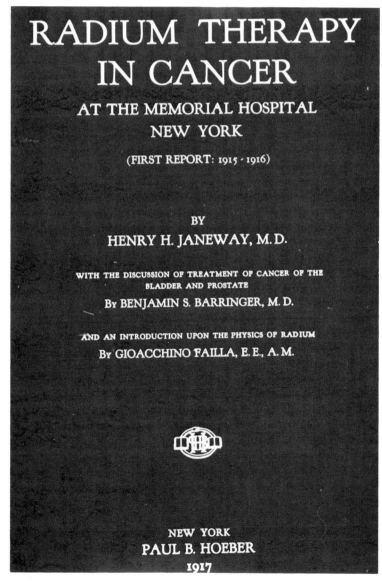

RADIUM THERAPY
IN CANCER

AT THE MEMORIAL HOSPITAL
NEW YORK

(FIRST REPORT: 1915 - 1916)

BY

HENRY H. JANEWAY, M.D.

WITH THE DISCUSSION OF TREATMENT OF CANCER OF THE
BLADDER AND PROSTATE

BY BENJAMIN S. BARRINGER, M.D.

AND AN INTRODUCTION UPON THE PHYSICS OF RADIUM

BY GIOACCHINO FAILLA, E.E., A.M.

NEW YORK
PAUL B. HOEBER
1917

FIGURE 2

In the 1930s, radium dosage tables based on the newly adopted unit of radiation, the *roentgen*, were developed by Paterson and Parker in Manchester and by Quimby at Memorial Hospital in New York City.

Quimby's research in biophysics set the basis for the comparison of biological and clinical effects of radium and also for protection from the undesirable effects of radiation (**Fig. 3**).

The term *Brachytherapy* was proposed for the first time by Forssel in 1931. Since then, various terms have been used to define the treatment by radionuclides, i.e., plesiotherapy, curietherapy, endocurietherapy, etc.

At first, the problems of radiation exposure intimidated many contemporary radiotherapists from using brachytherapy. Subsequently, however, lack of training opportunities in brachytherapy and "the mistaken belief that external-beam therapy could do anything and everything" (Hall, 1985), made radiotherapists believe that brachytherapy was obsolete.

Contributions made in the United States by Henschke in the 1950s, while he was practicing at Memorial Hospital drastically changed the image of brachytherapy (**Fig. 4**). These contributions included afterloading of the radioactive source and the introduction of Ir-192 as a substitute for Ra-226.

These developments, adopted by Pierquin and Chassagne in France, set the stage for the simultaneous rebirth of brachytherapy in the European continent.

Other advances made in the 1970s and 1980s in physics dosimetry, in computer technology, and in imaging techniques, such as CT and MRI, improved the accuracy of brachytherapy, improved the ability to delineate normal and neoplastic tissues, and facilitated the display of large amounts of information related to diagnosis and to radiation dose distribution.

In the 1930s to 1950s, the given dose in interstitial brachytherapy was usually defined according to the Paterson-Parker system. In the middle 1960s, the introduction of computers into medicine provided the first computerized radiation dose distributions. In the 1970s, two-dimensional iso-

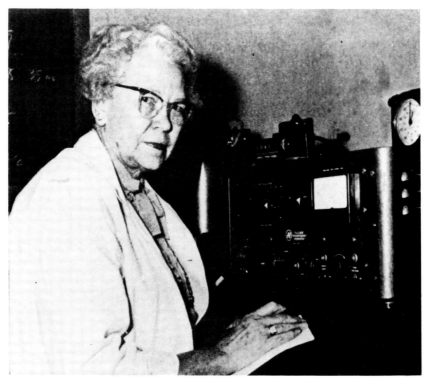

FIGURE 3. Edith Quimby, Ph.D. (1891–1982).

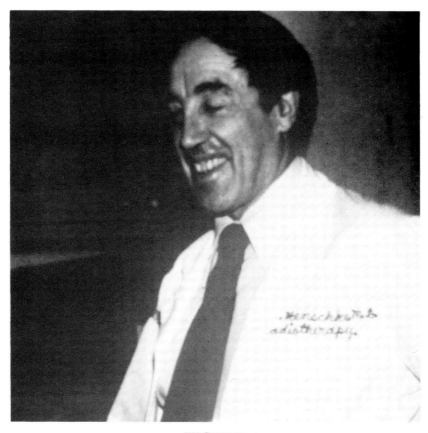

FIGURE 4

dose distributions were obtained, although they were initially drawn manually. As the technology improved, it took its current form, drawn by plotters. In the early 1980s, the isodose contour, corresponding to the measured dimensions of the target volume, was identified as MPD (matched peripheral dose). More recently, with the utilization of CT scans, a computerized three-dimensional dose distribution has become possible (**Fig. 5**).

The introduction of remote afterloading of radioactive sources and of low energy radionuclides (I-125) in Memorial Hospital in the early 1960s brought a marked reduction in radiation exposure to personnel and eased the fear associated with the use of radionuclides in brachytherapy (**Fig. 6**). The elimination of radiation exposure for most hospital personnel added to the convenience of the physician, but, more importantly, improved the care of the patients.

In the last three decades, following the introduction of afterloading, approximately 14,000 brachytherapy procedures have been performed at Memorial Hospital, providing the necessary information for this book (**Fig. 7**).

The ranks of brachytherapy in the 1980s are once more filled by enthusiastic, dynamic, well trained, and effective disciples, assuring a prominent position of the specialty in the war against cancer.

To this new *esprit de corps*, this book is dedicated.

REFERENCES

1. Abbe, R. Radium in surgery. *JAMA* 47:183–185, 1906.

2. Danlos, L. A. Sur l'action physiologique et therapeutique du radium. *Bull Sc Pharmacol* 9:65–74, 1904.

3. Quimby, E. H. The development of dosimetry in radium therapy. In: Hilaris, B. S. (ed.). *Afterloading: 20 Years of Experience, 1955–1975*. Proceedings of the Second International Symposium on Radiation Therapy, Memorial Sloan-Kettering Cancer Center, New York, 1975, pp. 1–6.

4. Paterson, R., and Parker, H. M. A dosage system for gamma ray therapy. *Br J Radiol* 7:592–612, 1934.

5. Quimby, E. H. The grouping of radium tubes in packs or plaques to produce the desired distribution of radiation. *Am J Roentgenol* 27:18, 1932.

6. Forssel, G. La lutte sociale contre le cancer. *J Radiol* 15:621–634, 1931.

7. Henschke, U. K., Hilaris, B. S., and Mahan, G. D. Afterloading in interstitial and intracavitary radiation therapy. *Am J Roentgenol Radium Ther Nucl Med* 90: 386–395, 1963.

8. Hall, E. J., and Lam, Y. M. The renaissance in low dose rate interstitial implant radiobiological consideration. *Front Radiat Ther Oncol* 12:21–34, 1978.

9. Hilaris, B. S., Nori, D., and Anderson, L. L. New approaches to brachytherapy. In: DeVita, V. A., Hellman, S., and Rosenberg, S. (eds.). *Important Advances in Oncology 1987*. Philadelphia: JB Lippincott Co., 1987. Part Two: Clnical Progress, Chapter 12:237–261.

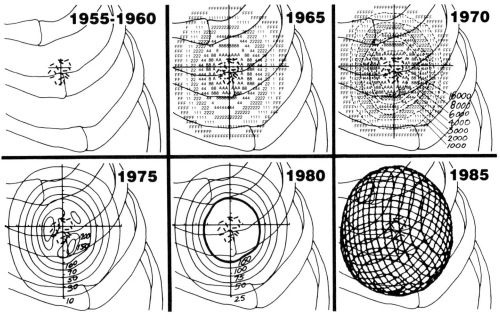

FIGURE 5

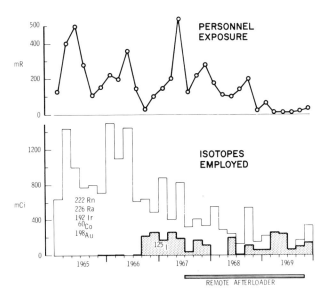

FIGURE 6

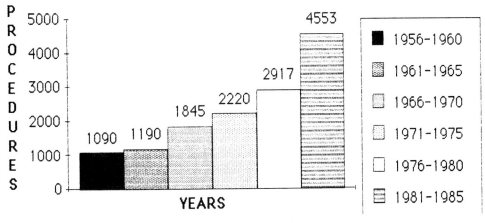

FIGURE 7

Acknowledgments

The list of individuals who assisted us in the preparation of this book is too lengthy to list individually, but it would be an omission if we did not acknowledge the help of my colleagues in the Departments of Surgery and Radiation Oncology at Memorial Sloan-Kettering Cancer Center, and our friends who provided us with the illustrations for the book. We would also like to thank Dina Mastoras and Fern Wright, who gave invaluable help in the preparation of this book.

Basil S. Hilaris, M.D., F.A.C.R.

Dattatreyudu Nori, M.D.

Lowell L. Anderson, Ph.D.

FIGURE	ACKNOWLEDGMENT
2-12, 13, and 16	Courtesy of Mick Radio-Nuclear Instruments, Inc., Bronx, New York.
5-10, 11, and 12	Courtesy of the International Commission on Radiation Units and Measurements (ICRU Report 38, 1985), Bethesda, Maryland.
6-1	Courtesy of Dr. Jatin Shah, Head and Neck Service. Memorial Sloan-Kettering Cancer Center, New York.
6-2	Fried, M.P. Cancer of the head and neck. Fig. 1, p. 33, April 1987. In: *Primary Care and Cancer.* Dominus Publishing Co., Williston Park, New York. Artwork: Harriet Phillips.
6-3	Courtesy of Dr. Louis Harrison, Brachytherapy Service. Memorial Sloan-Kettering Cancer Center, New York.
6-6 and 8, left	Modified from *MacAnatomy*, Vol. 1. Macmedia Publishers, Inc., Houston, Texas. Artwork: Dr. Robert Davis.
6-16, 17, and 18	Vikram, B., and Hilaris, B.S. A non-looping afterloading technique for interstitial implants of the base of the tongue. *Int. J. Radiat. Oncol. Biol. Phys.* 7:419–422, 1981.
6-20	Son, Y.H., and Kacinski, B.M. Therapeutic concepts of brachytherapy/megavoltage in sequence for pharyngeal wall cancers. Results of integrated dose therapy. Fig. 1 59:1268–1273, 1987.
8-1	Anatomy of the female breast (poster). Dominus Publishing Co., Williston Park, New York. Artwork: Harriet Phillips.
8-5 and 8	Shank, B. Breast preservation and brachytherapy. Fig. 1. *Endocurietherapy/Hyperthermia Oncol.* 2:S-17,24, 1986.
9-1, 3, 4, 5, and 6	Courtesy of Dr. Luis Linares. Brachytherapy Service, Memorial Sloan-Kettering Cancer Center, New York.
9-2, 7 (left & right), and 11	Hilaris, B.S., Shiu, M.H., Nori, D., et al. Limbsparing therapy for locally advanced soft tisssue sarcomas. Figs. 3,6,7,9. *Endocurietherapy/Hyperthermia Oncol.* I:17–21, 1985.
9-9 and 10	Courtesy of Dr. Man H. Shiu, Department of Surgery, Memorial Sloan-Kettering Cancer Center, New York.
10-1	Martini, N., Bains, M.S., McCormack, P.M., Kaiser, L.R., Burt, M.E., and Pomerantz, A.H. Results of surgical treatment for non-small cell carcinoma of the lung. Memorial Sloan-Kettering experience. Hoogstraen, A. (ed.), UICC: Standard Treatment Series. Treatment of Lung Tumors. Springer Verlag, Heidelberg, Germany (in press).
12-10, 11, and 12	Syed, A.M.N., et al. Temporary idirium-192 implantation in the management of carcinoma of the prostate. Figs. 1,2,3(A & B), pp. 83–91. In: Hilaris, B.S. and Batata, M.A. (eds.). Memorial Sloan-Kettering Cancer Center, New York. Brachytherapy Oncology Update 1983.
12-13 and 14	Courtesy of Dr. David Greenblatt. The Valley Hospital, Ridgewood, New Jersey.
13-1, 2, 3, and 4	Modified from *MacAnatomy*, Vol. 1. Macmedia Publishers, Inc., Houston, Texas. Artwork: Dr. Robert Davis.
14-1	Brown, G.S. Radiation therapy in the treatment of the cervix. In: Nori, D. and Hilaris, B.S. (eds.) *Radiation Therapy of Gynecological Cancer.* Alan R. Liss, Inc., New York. Fig. 1, pp. 101–113, 1987. Artwork: David Purnell.
14-7	Syed, A.M.N. and Puthawala, A. Interstitial intracavitary radiation. "Syed-Neblett" applicator in the treatment of cancer of the cervix. In: *Radiation Therapy of Gynecologic Cancer.* Nori, D. and Hilaris, B.S. (eds.). Alan R. Liss, Inc., New York, Fig. 1, pp. 297–307, 1987.
14-8 and 9 (left & right)	Syed, A.M.N., et al. Transperineal interstitial intracavitary "Syed-Neblett" applicator in the treatment of carcinoma of the uterine cervix. Figs. 3,5 and 6. *Endocurietherapy/Hyperthermia Oncol.* 2:1–13, 1986.
15-1	Nori, D. Principles of radiation therapy in the management of carcinoma of the endometrium. In: Nori, D. and Hilaris, B.S. (eds.). *Radiation Therapy of Gynecological Cancer.* Alan R. Liss, Inc., New York. Fig. 1, pp. 115–146, 1987. Artwork: David Purnell.
16-1	Nori, D. Principles of radiation therapy in the treatment of vaginal tumors. In: Nori, D. and Hilaris, B.S. (eds.). *Radiation Therapy of Gynecological Cancer.* Alan R. Liss, Inc., New York. Fig. 6, pp. 173–190, 1987.
17-1	Nori, D. Principles of radiotherapy in the treatment of cancer of the vulva. In: Nori, D. and Hilaris, B.S. (eds.). *Radiation Therapy of Gynecological Cancer.* Alan R. Liss, Inc., New York. Fig. 1, pp. 191–198, 1987.

PART I

Introduction

CHAPTER 1

Radionuclide Sources for Brachytherapy

EMISSION CHARACTERISTICS-1

Suitability of a given radionuclide for brachytherapy is determined largely by its half-life and by the type, energy, and abundance (number per decay event) of its emission. These characteristics are shown in **Table 1–1** for a number of nuclides for which either the utility in brachytherapy has been established in clinical practice or the potential for application is clearly discernible. Although historically of paramount importance in brachytherapy, radium has been omitted from the table because its long-lived alpha activity constitutes a significant broken-source health hazard and because equally effective but less hazardous radionuclides have long been available.

The half-life of a radionuclide must be long enough to permit shipping and implant preparation with an acceptable loss of source strength to decay, but it must also be short enough to permit source sizes sufficiently small for the intended application. The latter constraint arises primarily because source activity (decay rate) is directly proportional to the number of radioactive atoms present and inversely proportional to the half-life with which they decay; for a given activity requirement, a longer half-life requires a commensurately greater number of atoms, i.e., a larger source. Source size is also increased if the radionuclide is diluted with inactive atoms, either other isotopes of the same element (e.g., iridium atoms in an Ir-192 source) or a carrier material to diminish contamination risk (e.g., ceramic or glass for Cs-137 sources). Thus, half-lives for brachytherapy range from a few days to a few decades (for interstitial seeds) or a few centuries (for intracavitary sources). Between extremes, the half-life must be appropriate to the type of implant, i.e., permanent or temporary. For temporary implants, the longest half-life compatible with desired source size makes it easier to maintain a source inventory and makes reuse more feasible. For permanent implants, a half-life longer than a few days means a lower initial dose rate for treatment and, therefore, reduced exposure to staff during nursing and other patient-care procedures.

TABLE 1-1. Radionuclides for Brachytherapy

Nuclide	Symbol	Half-life	Emission Used in Therapy	Energy Spectrum of Prominent Emission(s) [Type: energy in keV (#/decay)....]	Penetration
Americium-241	^{241}Am	432 y	photon	gamma: 59.5(0.36)	HVL_{Pb} = 0.012 cm
Cesium-131	^{131}Cs	9.7 d	photon	X: 30–35(0.74)	HVL_{Pb} = 0.002 cm
Cesium-137	^{137}Cs	30.0 y	photon	gamma: 662(1.00	HVL_{Pb} = 0.6 cm
Cobalt-60	^{60}Co	5.26 y	photon	gamma: 1173(0.99) 1332(0.99)	HVL_{Pb} = 1.2 cm
Gold-198	^{198}Au	2.70 d	photon	gamma: 412(0.96)	HVL_{Pb} = 0.3 cm
Iodine-125	^{125}I	59.6 d	photon	X: 27–32(1.40).	HVL_{Pb} = 0.002 cm
Iridium-192	^{192}Ir	74.0 d	photon	gamma: 316 (0.83) 468 (0.48) 308 (0.30) 296 (0.29)	HVL_{Pb} = 0.3 cm
Palladium-103	^{103}Pd	17.0 d	photon	X: 20–23 (0.71)	
Samarium-145	^{145}Sm	340 d	photon	X: 38–45 (1.40) gamma: 61 (0.13)	HVL_{Pb} = 0.004 cm
Selenium-75	^{75}Se	118.5 d	photon	gamma: 265 (0.58) 136 (0.54) 280 (0.25) 121 (0.16) 401 (0.12)	HVL_{Pb} = 0.2 cm
Phosphorus-32	^{32}P	14.3 d	electron	beta: 1710 max (1.00)	$Range_{maxE}$ = 800 mg/cm^2
Ruthenium-106 Rhodium-106	^{106}Ru/ ^{106}Rh	367 d	electron	beta: 3550 max (0.68) 3050 max 2390 max (0.17)	$Range_{maxE}$ = 1800 mg/cm^2
Strontium-90/ Yttrium-90	^{99}Sr/ ^{90}Y	28.1 y	electron	beta: 2280 max (1.00)	$Range_{maxE}$ = 1100 mg/cm^2
Californium-252	^{252}Cf	2.65 y	neutron	fission: 2350 avg 3.8/f	HVL_{water} = 5 cm

EMISSION CHARACTERISTICS-2

For photon emitters, photon energies in the range 20 to 35 keV are preferable for interstitial work because they lead to relative dose distributions similar in the implanted region to those with higher energies but falling off more rapidly with distance in the region outside the implant (See **Fig. 1-1**). Energies in this range also permit effective reduction of staff exposure using the same methods (e.g., lead aprons) employed in diagnostic radiology. When beta emitters are used for brachytherapy, both the degree of dose confinement to the treatment region and the ease of staff protection are enhanced to the extent that the beta emission is free of associated gamma ray emission. Of those listed, P-32 and the Sr-90/Y-90 "mother–daughter" pair are pure beta emitters, and the Ru-106/Rh-106 pair involves only minor (0.34 per decay event) contamination with photons. For surface applications, the choice of beta emitter depends on the desired penetration depth, which (in milligrams per square centimeter) is closely the same in most materials. Cf-252 emits fission-spectrum neutrons for which the dose-versus-distance curve in tissue is similar to that of low energy photons; the effect of significant contamination with high energy gamma ray emission is diminished by the greater relative biological effect of the neutrons.

The radionuclides for which attenuation in water is shown in Fig. 1-1 are those that currently have found the widest application in brachytherapy (see **Table 1-2**). At Memorial Sloan-Kettering Cancer Center, I-125 seeds have been used extensively for permanent implants, and are now finding increasing application in temporary implants as well, including (with New York Hospital) eye plaques for ocular melanoma. Ir-192 in the form of seeds in ribbons has served for many years in temporary interstitial implants of many sites and as a cable-mounted source in high dose rate remote-afterloader treatments. Cs-137 has been found to be highly suitable for low dose rate intracavitary applications employing remote, as well as manual, afterloading.

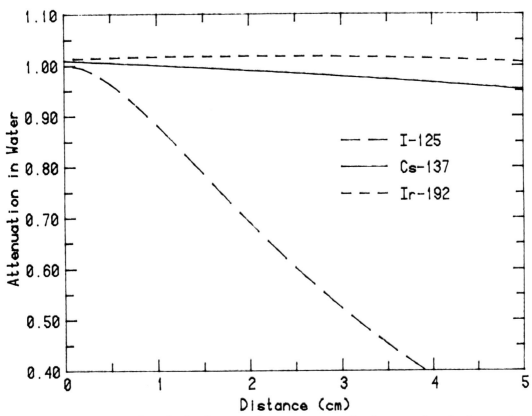

FIGURE 1-1. Ratio of air–kerma in water to air–kerma in air for point sources; Cs-137 and Ir-192 plots are best-fit polynomials from Meisberger et al. (1).

Table 1-2. Brachytherapy Radionuclides at Memorial Hospital

Nuclide	Average Photon Energy (MeV)	Half-Life	Application
I-125	0.028	59.6 d	Interstitial permanent Interstitial temporary Eye plaques
Ir-192	0.350	74.0 d	Interstitial temporary Remote afterloader intracavitary
Cs-137	0.662	30.0 y	Afterloading intracavitary

BRACHYTHERAPY QUANTITIES AND UNITS

The physical quantity of primary interest in radiation therapy is the *absorbed dose*, i.e., the energy absorbed per unit mass of tissue. Given in rads (1 rad = 100 ergs/g) until recently; the dose is now specified in Systeme International (SI) units of *gray*, for which the symbol abbreviation is Gy (1 Gy = 100 rad). To preserve the connection with the past, the preference is sometimes for *centigray* (1 cGy = 0.01 Gy = 1 rad).

Because of the relative ease of observing the ionization of air by radiation, by collecting the ions and determining the electrical charge, radiation has long been measured in terms of an air-ionization-based quantity, the *exposure*, for which the unit is the *roentgen* and the symbol is *R*. Historically, exposure was the antecedent of dose, and the units evolved in such a way that the dose to air per unit exposure (one way of expressing a quantity called W/e for air) is 0.87 cGy/R, not greatly different from unity. The dose to, say, muscle tissue per unit exposure for a given photon field is obtained by multiplying W/e by the mass energy absorption coefficient relative to air, which results in *f-factor* values close to 0.92 cGy/R for 20 to 35 keV photons (e.g., I-125) and 0.96 cGy/R for 150 keV to 2 MeV photons.

The quantity exposure is in the process of being displaced by a more general quantity, the *kerma*, which represents the energy transferred by uncharged ionizing particles (such as photons) to charged ionizing particles (such as secondary electrons) per unit mass of air or other material (2). Since kerma involves energy rather than ionization, its unit is the same as that of dose, i.e., the gray (Gy). For photon energies used in brachytherapy, where secondary electron ranges are short and bremsstrahlung production is negligible, kerma and dose are equal for practical purposes.

Activity, or decay rate, until recently specified for brachytherapy sources in millicurie units, where 1 millicurie = 3.7×10^7 decay event per second (the decay rate originally associated with 1 milligram of radium) is now specified by another SI unit, the *becquerel* (Bq), where 1 Bq = 1 decay event per second. *Cumulated activity*, the number of decay events having taken place in a certain time interval, may also be expressed in *millicurie-hours* (mCi h) (Table 1-3, 1-4).

For unencapsulated point sources, the photon output of a radionuclide has been characterized by its *exposure rate constant*, i.e., by the product of exposure rate and distance-squared per unit activity with units, typically, of roentgen centimeters-squared per millicurie-hours ($R\ cm^2/mCi\ h$). The successor to the exposure rate constant, of course, is the air–kerma rate constant, which is defined in an analogous manner.

TABLE 1-3. Brachytherapy Quantitites and Units

Quantity	Conventional Unit	Suggested SI Unit
Absorbed dose rate	rad/h	cGy/h
Exposure rate	R/h	—
Air–kerma rate	rad/h	cGy/h
Activity	mCi	MBq
Exposure rate constant	R cm^2/mCi h	—
Air–kerma rate constant	rad cm^2/mCi h	μG m^2/MBq H
Air–kerma strength	rad cm^2/h	μGy m^2/h
		cGy cm^2/h

TABLE 1-4. Photon Emission Rate Constants

Radionuclide	Exposure Rate Constant (R cm^2/mCi h)	Air-Kerma Rate Constant (μGy m^2/MBq h)
Cs-137	3.32	0.079
Ir-192	4.69	0.111
I-125	1.45	0.034

SOURCE STRENGTH SPECIFICATION

In view of the large fund of clinical experience with radium, brachytherapy sources of other radionuclides were often specified in units of *milligram radium equivalent* (mg Ra eq). *Equivalence* was defined in terms of exposure rate, i.e., a source had a strength of 1 mg Ra eq, if it produced the same exposure rate as a 1-mg radium source (with 0.5-mm Pt filtration) at the same distance in air, usually on the transverse axis of a linear source and far enough away that either source could be considered a point source. If the source's activity in millicuries was known, and if its encapsulation produced negligible interference with photon emission, the strength in milligram radium equivalents could be taken as the product of its activity in millicuries and the ratio of its exposure rate constant to that (8.25 R cm^2/mg h) of radium with 0.5 mm Pt filtration. This procedure, of course, was not valid for sources of low (20 to 35 keV) energy, for which attenuation in tissue would be much greater than for radium. Ir-192 and Cs-137 sources, typically, have been specified in milligram radium equivalents.

The equivalence concept was subsequently extended to allow specification of source strength in terms of *apparent activity*, defined as the activity of a point isotropic source, of the same radionuclide, which would duplicate the real source's exposure rate (or air–kerma rate), again at a transverse-axis distance far enough from source center that the inverse law is obeyed. Specification by apparent activity has been customary for I-125 seeds.

A brachytherapy dose calculation generally requires knowing the distance and orientation of the source with respect to the point of interest, together with the source strength and a composite multiplicative factor incorporating the dose per unit source strength and corrections for attenuation in the capsule and/or intervening tissue. The latter correction factor is given by F in the illustration (**Fig. 1-2**) for a point source. When source strength is given by apparent activity (defined by Eq. 1 in the illustration) the dose calculation involves multiplying the strength, A, by the air–kerma rate constant, Γ, to get a result, S (see Eq. 2). But A was obtained originally, via the calibration air–kerma rate measurement, by dividing by Γ (from Eq. 1). In practice, therefore, this method involves dividing and multiplying by the constant, Γ, which is evidently a fruitless exercise. Moreover, since the division may be performed by the source manufacturer and the multiplication by the user, the possibility that they may be using different values for the constant means a chance for error.

A much better approach has been developed by a task group of the American Association of Physicists in Medicine, which recommends specifying sources in terms of the *air–kerma strength*, defined as the product of air–kerma rate and distance-squared in free space, with the provision that the distance is always on the transverse axis and far enough away that the inverse square law holds, i.e., that the product will be independent of distance (3). This approach clearly makes the dose calculation more direct and less prone to error, as shown in Eq. 3 of Fig. 1-2.

$\dot{D}$ dose rate

$\dot{K}$ air–kerma rate

Γ air–kerma rate constant

A   apparent activity

F   product of air–kerma-to-dose conversion factor and tissue attenuation correction factor

d   distance from source

S   air–kerma strength

$$\text{For a point source, } S = \dot{K}\, d^2 = \Gamma A \tag{1}$$

INDIRECT: Source strength as apparent activity

$$\dot{D} = F\,\dot{K} = F\,\frac{\Gamma A}{d^2} = F\,\frac{\Gamma S/\Gamma}{d^2} = F\,\frac{S}{d^2} \tag{2}$$

DIRECT: Source strength as air–kerma strength

$$\dot{D} = F\,\dot{K} = F\,\frac{S}{d^2} \tag{3}$$

FIGURE 1-2. Direct versus indirect calculation of the dose rate for a point isotropic source.

IODINE-125

An I-125 atom decays by electron capture, i.e., capture by its nucleus of one of its inner-shell orbiting electrons. The decay is entirely to an excited state of Te-125, from which the transition to the ground state results, 7 percent of the time, in a 35-keV gamma ray. The other 93 percent of the time, this transition results, by *internal conversion*, in the removal of electrons from an atomic orbit, primarily from the inner, or *K*, orbit. Photon radiation from I-125 sources is thus primarily made up of characteristic Te-125 x-rays, which are emitted as electrons fall into the empty inner-orbit levels created by these two processes. I-125 is produced by thermal neutron irradiation of xenon gas enriched in Xe-124; the resulting Xe-125 atoms decay by electron capture to I-125 with a 17-hour half-life. The I-125 formed is removed during irradiation, to minimize the production of I-126, a contaminant activity with a 13-day half life.

I-125 seeds are furnished in two models, shown in a longitudinal cross section in **Fig. 1-3**(a,c). Although they have identical capsules, they differ greatly in radiographic visibility and significantly in photon energy spectrum. In the 6711 seed, the I-125 is deposited on the surface of a silver wire, which absorbs many of the emitted photons photoelectrically; a significant number of the resulting silver fluorescent photons, mainly at an energy of 22 keV, escape from the surface and contribute to the seed's photon emission (4). Average photon energy is lowered from about 28.5 keV to about 27.4 keV; the dose in water falls off discernibly faster with distance. The isodose contours shown in Fig. 1-3(b) for a 6711 seed of air–kerma 1.27 μGy m^2/h (1.00 mCi apparent activity) were calculated using a reference look-up table based on measurements by Ling and co-workers using thermoluminescent dosimeters (TLD) and silicon diodes (5). They illustrate the marked anisotropy of photon emission from the seed; the dose at 1 cm from seed center on the longitudinal axis of the seed is only about 40 percent that on the transverse axis.

Model 6711 seeds are used mainly for permanent implants where good radiographic visibility is required to permit dose evaluation. Their linear film images permit using a 2-D look up table to take anisotropy into account in dose calculations, if desired, even if seed orientation is somewhat random. If a single-dimension look up table is used, it is usual to account for anisotropy by multiplying the dose at all points by an average (over solid angle) anisotropy factor, 87 percent for the 6711 seed. Since a 6711 seed requires substantially more I-125 activity than a 6702 seed for a given air–kerma strength, 6711 seeds are used principally in relatively low-strength applications, 0.4 to 0.8 μGy m^2/h (0.3 to 0.6 mCi apparent activity).

Model 6702 seeds, with more efficient use of I-125 activity, are suitable for implants requiring fewer seeds of high activity, such as brain implants. In temporary implants of seeds in ribbons, radiographic visibility and orientation information are inferred from dummy ribbon images, and the lack of a marker is no disadvantage. Anisotropy and tissue attenuation, insofar as they affect dose distribution within the target region, are similar for 6702 and 6711 seeds.

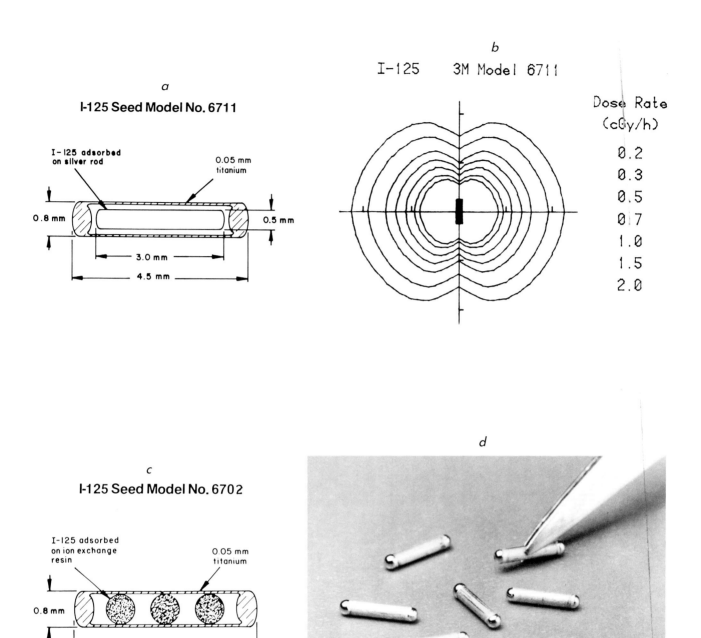

FIGURE 1-3. I-125 seed* characteristics: (a) 6711 *silver-wire* seed, (b) 6711 isodose rate contours, (c) 6702 *no-marker* seed, and (d) capsule appearance. *Medical-Surgical Division, 3M Company, St. Paul, MN.

IRIDIUM-192

The complexity of the Ir-192 photon energy spectrum (average energy 350 keV), evident from the "simplified" decay scheme shown in **Fig. 1-4**, may partially explain the wide variation among literature values of the exposure rate constant (6). This variation has increased the likelihood of error from failure to use the same value in calculations of source strength and dose and enhances the motivation for using air–kerma strength, thereby avoiding the needless involvement of the exposure rate constant (see Source Specification section). Ir-192 decays primarily by beta ray emission with a 74-day half life. It is formed by thermal neutron capture in reactor irradiation of natural iridium, from Ir-191 (37 percent abundant) together with Ir-194, a 19-hour half-life activity that arises from Ir-193 (63 percent abundant). In order to allow time for this competing activity to become insignificant, a supplier of clinical sources must delay shipping until about 2 weeks after irradiation of the preencapsulated iridium.

Ir-192 seeds are usually supplied as *ribbons*, intended for afterloading and, in which the seeds are press-fit at 1-cm intervals, in a thin nylon tube (as in the "dummy" ribbon of **Fig. 1-5**). **Figure 1-6** shows a same-film radiograph and autoradiograph of an array of Ir-192 ribbons. Individual seeds have a diameter of 0.5 mm and a length of 3.0 mm. One type of commercially available seed* employs an inner core of Pt–Ir (30-percent Ir) alloy 0.1 mm in diameter and 2.4 mm long, which is doubly encapsulated in stainless steel (7). In another,[†] the core is of Pt–Ir (10-percent Ir) alloy and the sheath (0.1 mm thick) is of platinum (8). An alternative source geometry is Ir-192 wire,[‡] with a core of Pt–Ir (25-percent Ir) and a 0.1-mm Pt sheath with an outer diameter of either 0.3 mm or 0.6 mm (9); the thinner wire, with a plastic sheath, is used for afterloading in larger-diameter catheters, while the thicker wire is sufficiently rigid for direct insertion in tissue with the aid of slotted steel guides. Encapsulation by either 0.1-mm platinum or 0.2-mm stainless steel suffices for the near-complete absorption of Ir-192 beta rays (maximum energy 0.67 MeV) except at cut ends of seeds or wires, where the effective absorber thickness may be smaller.

Ir-192 photon energies are high enough that exponential attenuation in water is almost exactly compensated by scattering buildup and the product of dose rate and distance squared is nearly constant (see Fig. 1-1) at distances less than 5 cm. In addition, since Ir-192 seeds are small enough to be good geometrical approximations to point sources and to give rise to only minimal anisotropy (at least in the case of stainless steel seeds), the practice of calculating dose in muscle tissues, for example, as the product of air–kerma rate in air and a constant ratio (about 1.10) of mass energy absorption coefficients should involve errors less than 2 to 3 percent at distances within 5 cm of the implanted region.

Somewhat larger (but still small) Ir-192 sources are appropriate for high-dose-rate remote afterloaders. **Figure 1-7** shows a cable-mounted intersti-

---

*Best Industries, Inc., Springfield, VA.
*Rad/Irid, Inc., Landover, MD.
[†]Alpha-Omega Services, Inc., Paramount, CA.
[‡]Amersham Corporation, Buckinghamshire, England.

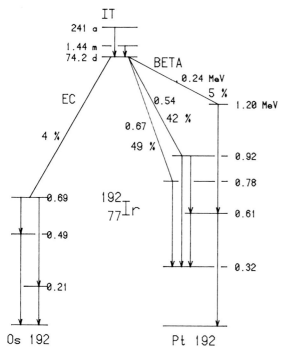

FIGURE 1-4. Ir-192 decay scheme in which branching pathways of less than 5 percent per decay have been omitted.

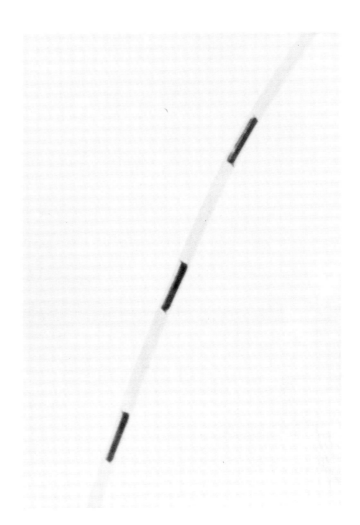

FIGURE 1-5. Dummy ribbon, for localization purposes, showing arrangement of Ir-192 seeds.

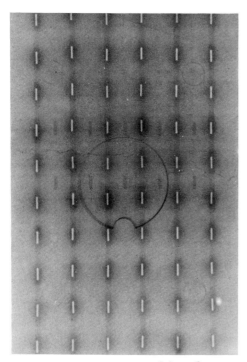

FIGURE 1-6. Combined radiograph and autoradiograph of Ir-192 seeds in ribbons.

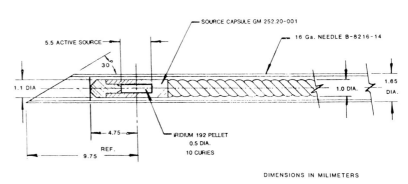

DIMENSIONS IN MILIMETERS

FIGURE 1-7. Assembled source capsule and open capsule (four iridium pellets and end cap) of cable-mounted Ir-192 source* used with Gamma Med IIi interstitial remote afterloader.

*Mallinckrodt Diagnostica (Holland) B. V., and Isotopen-Technik Dr. Sauerwein GMBH, Haan, West Germany.

13

tial source used in the Gamma Med IIi afterloader.* This source with a capsule diameter of 1 mm and an active length of 5 mm, can be positioned sequentially for programmable dwell-times at uniformly spaced points along one or more needles or catheters in treatment locations.

CESIUM-137

Cesium-137 is produced by fission in nuclear reactors. It decays by beta emission to Ba-137, 7 percent of the time directly and 93 percent of the time through a metastable state having a 2.5-minute half-life. A 662-keV monoenergetic photon is emitted in the *isomeric transition* of this Ba-137 metastable state.

With a half-life of 30 years, Cs-137 is well suited for intracavitary sources, where its specific activity (even when diminished for protection reasons by inactive, chemically inert carrier material) is more than adequate for low dose rate ($<$60 cGy/h) protocols. Thus, in commercially available sources of the design shown in **Fig. 1-8**(a), Cs-137-labeled ceramic microspheres are doubly encapsulated in stainless steel, with an outer-cylinder length of 20 mm and diameter of 3.1 mm.† Specific activities sufficiently high to permit a tissue dose rate of 320 cGy/h at a distance of 1 cm from the source center along the transverse axis. The isodose contours shown in Fig. 1-8(b) represent measured values of dose rate for a source having an air-kerma strength of 72 μGy m^2/h (10 mg Ra eq) (10,11). For distances of 2 cm and farther from the source center, the contours do not differ greatly from spherical in shape.

A further brachytherapy application of Cs-137 is in remote afterloading. The Selectron‡ low dose rate remote afterloader, for example, makes use of up to 48 identical spherical sources of the type shown in the cutaway drawing of **Fig. 1-9.** Although the radionuclide is incorporated in a glass matrix in this instance, source strengths as high as 116 μGy m^2/h (40 mCi) are readily available.

---

*Isotopen-Technik Dr. Sauerwein GMBH, Haan, West Germany, and Mick Radio-Nuclear Instruments, Bronx, NY.
†Medical-Surgical Division, 3M Company, St. Paul, MN.
‡Nucletron Corporation, Leersum, The Netherlands.

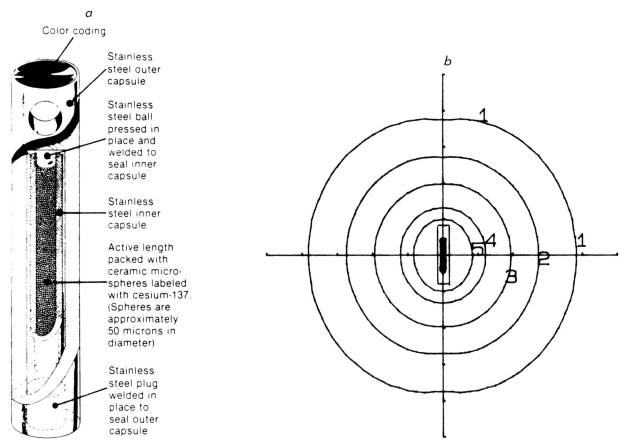

FIGURE 1-8. Cs-137 intracavitary tube source for manual afterloading: (a) cutaway view of source construction*, (b) isodose rate contours in (muscle) tissue, corresponding to 5, 10, 20, 50, and 100 cGy/h, for a source with a 1-cm active length. *Medical Surgical Division, 3M Company, St. Paul, MN.

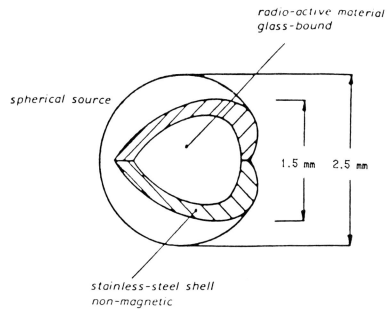

FIGURE 1-9. Spherical Cs-137 source for remote afterloading.*
*Amersham, Buckinghamshire, England, and Nucletron Corporation, Leersum, The Netherlands.

NEW OR EXPERIMENTAL RADIONUCLIDE SOURCES-1

The advent of nuclear reactors and the availability of artificial radionuclides stimulated a vigorous effort to identify radionuclides that might be particularly well-suited for brachytherapy. One of the more unusual candidate nuclides proposed was *californium-252* (Cf-252), a neutron emitter for which the rationale, for external beam neutrons, involves countering the radio-resistance of hypoxic cells with radiation for which the oxygen-enhancement ratio is lower.

Ribbons incorporating Cf-252 seeds of the type shown in **Fig. 1-10** were used at Memorial Sloan-Kettering Cancer Center in the 1970s for a small series of temporary interstitial implants to assess the feasibility of neutron brachytherapy techniques (12). The Memorial study was part of a U.S. Department of Energy program conceived in 1965 to evaluate Cf-252 for brachytherapy—a program that ultimately involved 18 institutional participants in the United States, England, and Japan (13). Cf-252 decays with a 2.65-year half-life, emitting fission-spectrum neutrons with an average energy of 2.35 MeV together with a significant number of gamma rays, both from fission events and fission products. In the interstitial seed shown in the figure, the core consists of a ceramic-metal (cermet) mixture of Cf-252 oxide and palladium, and the Pt (10-percent Ir) encapsulation is designed to limit the combined beta ray and gamma ray dose to one-third the effective dose from neutrons (using an RBE of 6.0) (14). Dosimetry studies at several institutions established single-source reference data indicating a near-source neutron dose rate per unit source strength of 2.3 cGy cm^2/μg h in muscle tissue; source strength specification is in micrograms (μg) of Cf-252 (15). Beta rays do not penetrate the capsule of intracavitary Cf-252 sources, for which the gamma ray dose at 0.5 cm is lower by another factor of three. Clinical trials of Cf-252 are currently in progress at several institutions in the United States, Japan, and the U.S.S.R. (16).

Photons from *americium-241* (Am-241) are of sufficiently low energy (60 keV) that they are effectively attenuated by relatively light shields and of sufficiently high abundance that dose rate distributions comparable to those from Cs-137 are possible (refer to Table 1-1). These characteristics suggest the feasibility of dose-distribution shaping with internal shields, as well as the simplified radiation protection of staff, and, together with the long half-life of Am-241, make this radionuclide an attractive alternative for intracavitary brachytherapy and have motivated developmental studies by Nath et al. (17).

^{252}Cf NEUTRON SOURCE (SEED) ALC-P4C
Nominal Dimensions

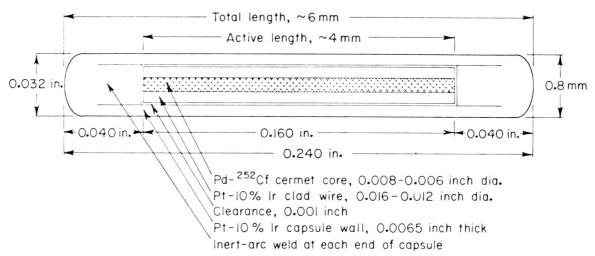

FIGURE 1-10. **Cf-252 afterloading seed for interstitial neutron therapy.***
*United States Department of Energy, Savannah River Laboratory, Aiken, SC.

NEW OR EXPERIMENTAL RADIONUCLIDE SOURCES-2

In a recent review of research directions in brachytherapy (18); the need was set forth for a low-energy photon emitter to use in permanent interstitial implants of rapidly proliferating tumors, i.e., an emitter having a half-life shorter than that of I-125. Such an emitter is *palladium-103* (Pd-103) (17-day half-life), which is now being proposed* for clinical use in a capsule (see **Fig. 1-11**) of similar dimensions as an I-125 seed. The stable isotope Pd-102, uniformly distributed throughout aluminum cylinders at each end of the seed's interior, is converted to Pd-103 by thermal neutron capture when the entire seed is irradiated after assembly. Pd-103 decays, by electron capture, to a metastable state (56-minute half-life) of Rh-103, whose characteristic x-rays of 20 to 23 keV are emitted as electrons fill vacancies resulting from either the decay itself or internal conversion of gamma rays. Although lightweight end-closures minimize photon absorption, lower photon energy results in a solid-angle-averaged anisotropy (83 percent) that is comparable to that of I-125 seeds and in somewhat more compact dose distributions in tissue.

A further need expressed in the previously mentioned review was for a radionuclide with low photon energy and long half-life for ophthalmic applicators and other temporary implants for which reuse may be desirable (18). A promising candidate for this application is *samarium-145* (Sm-145), which is formed by neutron activation from samarium enriched in Sm-144 and which decays by electron capture to promethium-145, also radioactive, with a 17.7-year half-life, which decays by electron capture to (stable) neodymium-145. Although the 340-day half-life and 38- to 45-keV x-ray energies of Sm-245 suggest possible specific-activity and self-absorption constraints on source strength, titanium-encapsulated seeds (4.5-mm long by 0.8-mm diameter) have been fabricated with air–kerma strengths of about 3.5 μGy m^2/h (equivalent to 2.8 mCi apparent of I-125); an experimental eye plaque has been fabricated as well (19). An interesting feature of Sm-145 is the possibility of enhancing its radiation dose by administering iodinated deoxyuridine, a thymidine analog; Sm-145 photon energies fall just above the *K* absorption edge (33.2 keV) of iodine where the interaction probability is near maximum (19).

---

*Theragenics Corporation, Atlanta, GA.

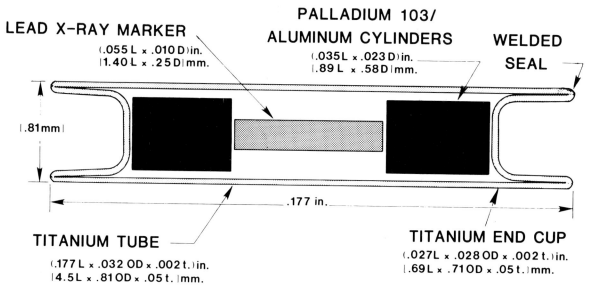

LEAD X-RAY MARKER
(.055 L x .010 D) in.
(1.40 L x .25 D) mm.

PALLADIUM 103/
ALUMINUM CYLINDERS
(.035L x .023 D) in.
(.89 L x .58D) mm.

WELDED
SEAL

(.81mm)

.177 in.

TITANIUM TUBE
(.177 L x .032 OD x .002 t.) in.
(4.5 L x .81 OD x .05 t.) mm.

TITANIUM END CUP
(.027L x .028 OD x .002 t.) in.
(.69L x .71 OD x .05 t.) mm.

FIGURE 1-11.   Pd-103 seed for interstitial brachytherapy.*
***Theragenics Corporation, Atlanta, GA**

CALIBRATION

The core of the rationale for specifying sources in terms of air–kerma strength is the fact that the National Bureau of Standards (NBS) calibrations for major brachytherapy sources (Cs-137, Ir-192, and I-125) are based on measurements of ionization in air, i.e., currently on exposure rate, from which the air–kerma rate differs, at brachytherapy energies, only by the constant factor, 0.87 cGy/R. The NBS exposure rate standard for Cs-137 sources was established by careful measurements at 50 cm along the transverse axis from stainless-steel encapsulated sources (13.5-mm long × 7.1-mm diameter) by using spherical graphite ionization chambers that were 20.7 mm in diameter in open-air geometry (20). Sources submitted for calibration are compared by substitution at an appropriate distance from a track-mounted 2.5-L aluminum spherical chamber designed for routine measurements, with a "working standard" source of similar same strength (20). Overall uncertainty in the calibration is given as 3.2 percent.

Spherical graphite chambers of slightly larger volume (50 cc) were used in the NBS calibration of Ir-192 seeds; open air measurements were performed at 0.5 m and 1.0 m from an array of seeds (21). Calibrations for both platinum and stainless-steel seeds were transferred to a reentrant spherical aluminum chamber (see **Fig. 1-12**) in which individual seeds submitted by users are inserted for measurement. Small variations in photon emission anisotropy and in chamber angular response patterns result in a chamber calibration factor (source strength per unit chamber current) 3 percent higher for platinum than for stainless-steel seed construction. Calibration uncertainty for Ir-192 is estimated to be 2.0%.

In the case of I-125 seeds, the NBS calibration made use of a standard free-air ionization chamber (for 20 to 100 kV x-rays) with measurements at 0.25 m and 0.5 m from an array of seeds mounted in a cylindrical aluminum collimator having an identical photon port at 180 degrees to avoid backscattering (22). Calibrations for both 6711 and 6702 seeds were transferred to the same spherical aluminum chamber used for Ir-192 seeds, modified only by replacing the original brass source-holder tube with one of aluminum. The chamber calibration factor for the 6711 (silver-wire) seed was 20 percent higher than that for the 6702 (no-marker) seed, reflecting a very significant difference in the convolution of seed-emission and chamber-response angular variations. Stated calibration uncertainties are 2.1 percent for the 6711 seed and 1.5 percent for the 6702 seed (22).

Because of the strong dependence of reentrant chamber sensitivity on source construction, NBS calibrations for Ir-192 and I-125 are specific to certain source designs. When sources of other designs (or of other radionuclides) are to be used, the basic measurement of air–kerma strength must be undertaken for the source type of interest. A relationship to NBS standards, though one step removed, is nonetheless achievable by using ionization chambers with calibrations traceable to NBS. **Figure 1-13** shows the arrangement of apparatus, for example, for calibrating a Gamma Med II remote afterloader Ir-192 source which is cable-mounted and stainless-steel encapsulated with active dimensions of 1.2 mm × 1.2 mm. A 3-cc Shonka-Wyckof chamber (23) of air-equivalent conductive plastic is being used at a distance of 40 cm from the source.

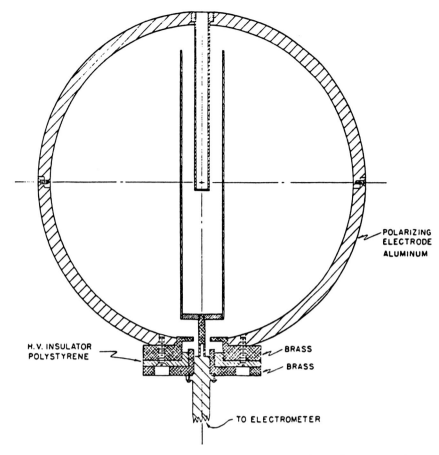

FIGURE 1-12. Aluminum reentrant chamber used at the National Bureau of Standards for measurement of Ir-192 and I-125 seeds (from Ref. 22, used by permission).

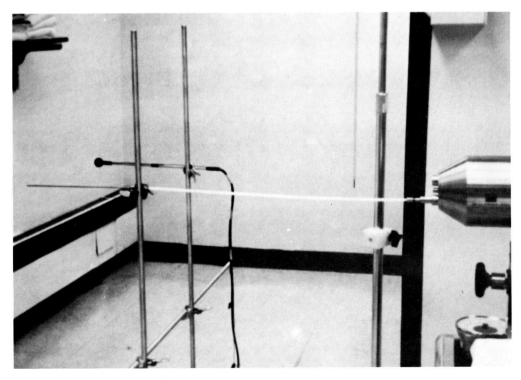

FIGURE 1-13. Measurement geometry for calibration of Gamma Med II remote afterloader Ir-192 source.

QUALITY ASSURANCE

In the local hospital, it is the cylindrical reentrant ionization chamber, i.e., the *well chamber*, that has been recommended for quality assurance checks of brachytherapy source strength (24). **Figure 1-14** depicts a well-chamber designed expressly for this purpose at the Radiological Physics Center (RPC) (25). More widely available are well-chamber instruments used as *dose calibrators* in nuclear medicine departments, an example of which is shown in **Fig. 1-15** (26). For the RPC chamber, a plastic source holder with centering spacers is provided to position a source (or ribbon of sources) reproducibly on the axis of a relatively narrow channel, whereas a lightweight (open) cylindrical frame is used to center sources in the wider well of the nuclear-medicine type chamber.

It is recommended that a representative single source, of the radionuclide and source design to be used, be sent to the NBS (or a secondary standards laboratory) for calibration. The calibrated source then serves to provide calibration factors (source strength per unit instrument response) for one or more well chambers. A second chamber calibration affords a valuable resource if the primary chamber result is questioned. In transferring the calibration to the local-hospital chamber, it is important that the source position in the chamber be central and carefully determined. If clinical sources, such as seeds in ribbons, are to be checked at axial positions other than the calibration reference point, it is necessary that the relative chamber response be determined at all such points.

A long-lived reference source is essential for quality assurance checks of radionuclides, such as Ir-192 and I-125, having relatively short half-lives. Preferably the reference source strength should produce roughly the same chamber ion current as the sources to be checked in order to avoid the uncertainties related to recombination effects or the use of different instrument scales. The "standard" source should be compared with the reference source by substitution within the chamber using identical instrument settings both before and after its source strength is determined by the standards laboratory. A *chamber-calibration factor* may then be defined as the source strength per unit chamber response, with proper operation verified by obtaining the expected response to the reference source. Alternatively, these data may be used to determine the constant of proportionality between source strength and the clinical-source–reference-source ratio of chamber responses; this method might be preferred if the chamber cavity is open to ambient air because temperature and pressure corrections, otherwise necessary in checks of clinical sources, would thereby be avoided. In either method, reference-source readings are required at the time clinical sources are checked.

It should be kept in mind that each chamber-calibration factor is valid only for a given source design and a given radionuclide.

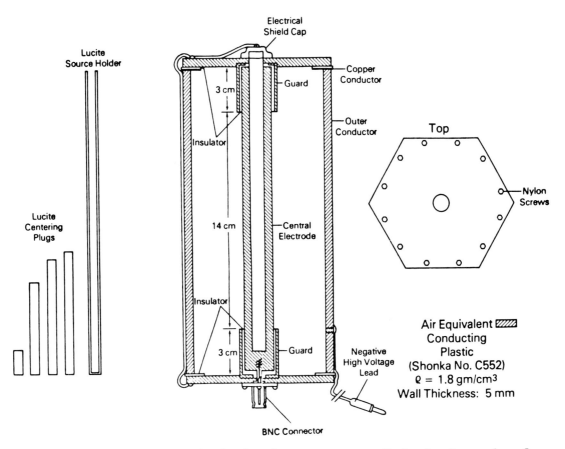

FIGURE 1-14. Radiological Physics Center well ionization chamber (from Ref. 25, used by permission).

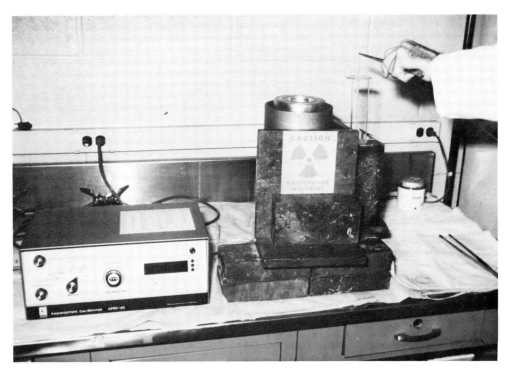

FIGURE 1-15. Dose calibrator well ionization chamber* used for brachytherapy source quality assurance checks.
*CPRC-20 Radio-isotope Calibrator, Capintec, Inc., Montvale, N.J.

RADIATION PROTECTION

Just as the gray is replacing the rad (1 Gy = 100 rad) as the unit of dose in radiation physics, another SI unit, the *sievert* (Sv) is replacing the rem (1Sv = 100 rem) as the unit of dose equivalent in radiation protection (26). The suggested convention during the transition period is to give each stated value a second time, in parentheses, in the old (rem) units.

Storage and handling of brachytherapy sources should be guided broadly by the dose-limiting recommendations of the National Council on Radiation Protection and Measurements, e.g., a maximum permissible whole body dose equivalent of 50 mSv (5 rem) in any 1 year for occupationally exposed persons and 5 mSv (0.5 rem) in any 1 year for occasionally exposed persons (27). For transport within the hospital, shielding containers for higher-energy sources, such as Cs-137 and Ir-192, should employ a combination of an appropriate thickness of lead together with spatial separation by long handles (see Table 1-1 and **Fig. 1-16**), whereas for low energy sources, such as I-125 seeds, more compact containers of brass or stainless steel generally suffice. A reasonable criterion for storage and transport containers is that measurable surface levels not exceed 100 μSv/h = (10 mrem/h). Preparation of materials for I-125 implants is frequently facilitated by transparent lead acrylic (see **Fig. 1-17**).

Measurements of each implanted patient at the proximal body surface and at 1m from the implant center should be recorded, with appropriate demographic information, in a permanent log. The data should also be used to complete "radioactive precautions" tags to be affixed to the patient's chart, bed, door of room, and wrist (**Fig. 1-18**). A level greater than 20 μSv/h (2 mrem/h) at 1 m should be supplemented by measurements in adjoining rooms and may lead to a decision to use a bedside shield. It is important that implanted patients be provided basic information and reassurance regarding radiation precautions, with special attention to patients being discharged with implanted radioactivity. An effective educational program for the nursing staff is essential to assure undiminished care of the implanted patient, proper management of visitors, and appropriate response to unusual situations (28).

Personnel monitoring is required for all staff who might receive a significant fraction, say one-quarter, of the maximum permissible dose. In addition to a whole-body film badge, persons whose work requires preparation or manipulation of implant sources are supplied and advised to wear a wrist film badge and a finger TLD (see **Fig. 1-19**). A badge-exchange interval of 1 month is recommended.

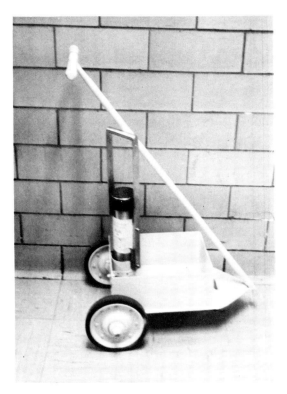

FIGURE 1-16. Lead shield container and cart used to transport Cs-137 intracavitary sources to patient's room for afterloading.

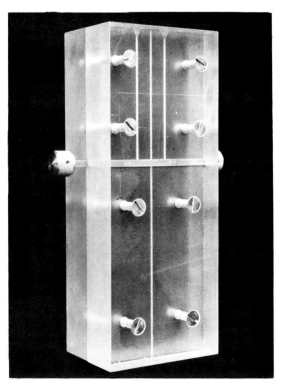

FIGURE 1-17. Seed feeder of lead-acrylic plastic* (1.5-mm Pb equivalent) for compressed-air loading of I-125 seeds and spacers in temporary-implant ribbons.
*Victoreen Nuclear Associates, Carle Place, NY.

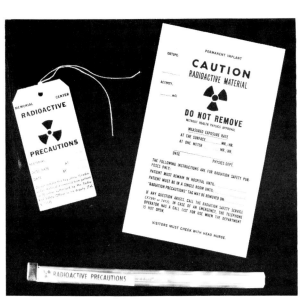

FIGURE 1-18. Precaution tags for implanted patients.

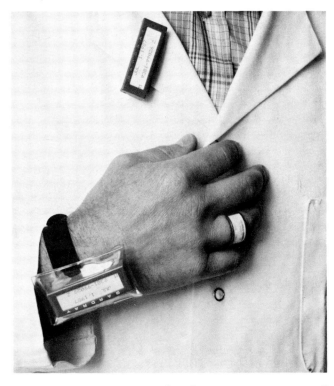

FIGURE 1-19. Brachytherapy personnel exposure monitors.

REFERENCES

1. Meisberger, L. L., Keller, R. J., and Shalek, R. J. The effective attenuation in water of the gamma rays of gold-198, iridium-192, cesium-137, radium-226 and cobalt-60. *Radiology* 90:953–957, 1968.

2. International Commission on Radiation Units and Measurements (ICRU). Radiation quantities and units, ICRU Report #33. Washington DC: ICRU, 1980: 25.

3. Nath, R., Anderson, L., Jones, D., Ling, C., Loevinger, R., Williamson, J., and Hanson, W. Specification of Brachytherapy Source Strength (AAPM Report No. 21), A Report of Task Group 32, Radiation Therapy Committee, American Association of Physicists in Medicine. New York: American Institute of Physics, 1987, 21 pp.

4. Ling, C. C., Yorke, E. D., Spiro, I. J., Kubiatowicz, D., and Bennett, D. Physical dosimetry of ^{125}I seeds of a new design for interstitial implant. *Int J Radiat Oncol Biol Phys* 9:1747–1752, 1983.

5. Ling, C. C., Schell, M. C., Yorke, E. D., Palos, B. B., Kubiatowicz, D. O. Two dimensional dose distribution of I-125 seeds. *Med Phys* 12:652–655, 1985.

6. Glasgow, G. P., and Dillman, L. T. Specific x-ray constant and exposure rate constant of ^{192}Ir. *Med Phys* 6:49–52, 1979.

7. Suthanthiran, K. Interstitial implant technique using iridium-192. In: Shearer, D. R. (ed.), *Recent Advances in Brachytherapy Physics*, Medical Physics Monograph No. 7, New York: American Institute of Physics, 1981, pp. 49–54.

8. Stephens, S. O. ^{192}Ir production quality assurance. In: Shearer, D. R. (ed.), *Recent Advances in Brachytherapy Physics*, Medical Physics Monograph No. 7, New York: American Institute of Physics, 1981, pp. 72–76.

9. Dutreix, A., Marinello, G., and Wambersie, A. *Dosimetrie en Curie-Therapy* Paris: Masson, 1982, p. 277.

10. Mohan, R., Ding, I. Y., Martel, M. K., Anderson, L. L., Nori, D. Measurements of radiation dose distributions for shielded cervical applicators. *Int J Radiat Oncol Biol Phys* 11:861–868, 1985.

11. Drozdoff, V., Thomason, C. L., and Anderson, L. L. 3D Cs-137 dose distributions for cervix applicator shielded ovoid (Abstr.). *Med Phys* 10:536, 1983.

12. Vallejo, A., Hilaris, B. S., Anderson, L. L. ^{252}Cf for interstitial implantation: a clinical study at Memorial Hospital. *Int J Radiat Oncol Biol Phys* 2:731–737, 1977.

13. Stoddard, D. H. Historical review of californium-252 discovery and development. *Nucl Sci Applications* 2:189–199, 1986.

14. Permar, P. H. ^{252}Cf neutron sources for interstitial after-loading. *Int J Radiat Oncol Biol Phys* 1:1003–1009, 1976.

15. Anderson, L. L. Cf-252 physics and dosimetry. *Nucl Sci Applications* 2:273–281, 1986.

16. Maruyama, Y. Californium-252: new radioisotope for human cancer therapy. *Endocuriether Hyperthermia Oncol* 2:171–187, 1986.

17. Nath, R., and Gray, L. Dosimetric studies on prototype ^{241}Am sources for brachytherapy. *Int J Radiat Oncol Biol Phys* 13:897–905, 1987.

18. Phillips, T. L., Fu, K. K., Goffinet, D., Ling, C., Anderson, L., and Suntharalingam, N. *Brachytherapy Cancer Treatment Symposia* 1:119–126, 1984.

19. Fairchild, R. G., Kalef-Ezra, J., Packer, S., Wielopoloski, L., Laster, B. H., Robertson, J. S., Mausner, L., and Kanellitsis, C. Samarium-145; a new brachytherapy source. *Phys Med Biol* 32:847–858, 1987.

20. Loftus, T. P. Standardization of cesium-137 gamma-ray sources in terms of exposure units (roentgens). *J Res Nat Bur Stand* 74A:1–6, 1970.

21. Loftus, T. P. Standardization of iridium-192 gamma-ray sources in terms of exposure. *J Res Nat Bur Stand* 85:19–25, 1980.

22. Loftus, T. P. Exposure standardization of iodine-125 seeds used for brachytherapy. *J Res Nat Bur Stand* 89:295–303, 1984.

23. Boag, J. W. Ionization chambers. In: Attix, F. H., and Roesch, W. C. (eds.): *Radiation Dosimetry, Second Edition.* volume II: Instrumentation, New York: Academic Press, 1966, pp. 1–72.

24. Hanson, W. F., Anderson, L. L., Ling, C. C., Loevinger, R., and Strubler, K. A. Brachytherapy. In: Physical aspects of quality assurance in radiation therapy (AAPM Report No. 13). New York, American Institute of Physics, 1984, pp. 38–47.

25. Berkeley, L. W., Hanson, W. F., and Shalek, R. J. Discussion of the characteristics and results of measurements with a portable well ionization chamber for calibration of brachytherapy sources. In: Shearer D. R. (ed.): *Recent Advances in Brachytherapy Physics*, Medical Physics Monograph No. 7. New York: American Institute of Physics, 1981, pp. 38–48.

26. National Council on Radiation Protection and Measurements (NCRP). *SI Units in Radiation Protection and Measurements*, NCRP Report No. 82. Washington, DC: NCRP, 1985, p. 64.

27. National Council on Radiation Protection and Measurements (NCRP). *Protection Against Radiation from Brachytherapy Sources*, NCRP Report No. 40. Washington, DC: NCRP, 1972, p. 65.

28. Leahy, L., St. Germain, J., and Varricchio, C. *The Nurse and Radiotherapy*. St. Louis: Mosby 1978, p. 240.

CHAPTER 2

Brachytherapy Instruments

INTERSTITIAL BRACHYTHERAPY INSTRUMENTS

Permanent Implantation

The use of single source inserters is satisfactory for small planar permanent implants, especially superficial tumors, where the desired implantation pattern can be clearly marked on the skin. Since most intrathoracic and intraabdominal tumors require volume implants with many seeds, the individual source inserters crowd the field, are difficult to position in an orderly fashion, and make many more punctures than necessary. Special implantation instruments, therefore, have been designed to allow more accurate and fairly rapid implementation of the permanent implantation technique.

"Mick" Applicator (Fig. 2-1).   The preparation of this applicator prior to surgery is important. Many difficulties and inconveniences will be avoided by carefully following the manufacturer's instructions. As with any other new equipment, it is essential to become acquainted with its features and functions before using it. The set supplied by the manufacturer (Mick Radio-Nuclear Instruments, Inc., Bronx, NY) includes a magazine for loading the radioactive sources, hypodermic stainless-steel needles, a stainless-steel ruler, and several other accessories, in addition to the applicator. A stainless-steel caliper is useful for tumor measurements (**Fig. 2-2**). A commercially available V-block is useful for loading sources into the cartridge (**Fig. 2-3**).

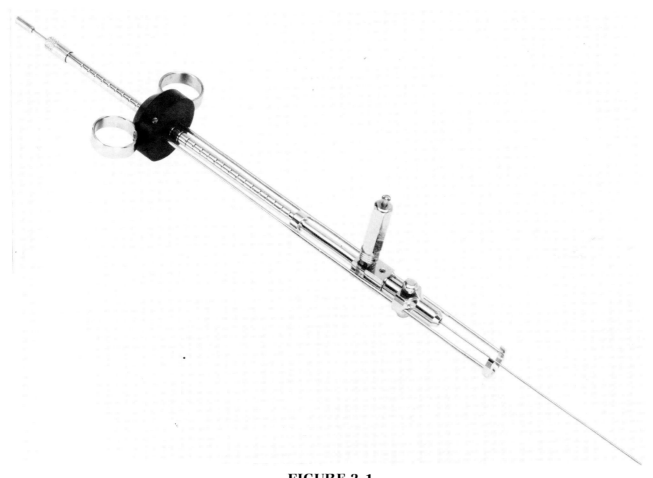

FIGURE 2-1

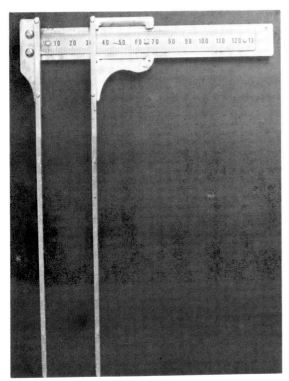

FIGURE 2-2

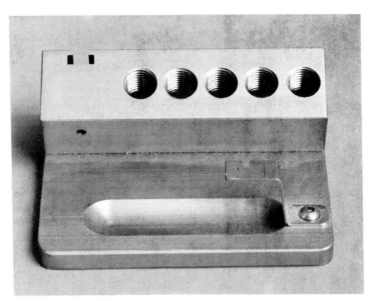

FIGURE 2-3

Preparation. The first step in preparing this instrument for implantation of I-125 seeds is loading the magazines. Magazines are stored in the magazine holder of the stainless-steel tray and may be removed by unscrewing counterclockwise (clockwise for storage). Seeds that are under or oversized should not be used because they could cause jamming of the magazine or applicator. When the cartridge is loaded to capacity, the magazine head plunger is inserted into the cartridge slot and turned clockwise with slight downward pressure until it stops. The magazine is then ready for implantation and can be put back into the steel tray. The magazine holder is provided with five holes to store five magazines. The instrument is provided with a ratchet mechanism and gauge to facilitate placement of seeds at desired intervals and depths. Needles are withdrawn in 5-mm steps and seeds are manually ejected, using a stylet, into the tumor. Each needle simply slips into the needle receptor and is firmly held in place by retainer springs. In order to remove the needle, two buttons located opposite each other on the needle receptor must be depressed simultaneously. This feature reduces the chance of accidental disengagement of the needle.

In addition to the standard-size Mick applicator for 15 cm needles, there are models that accommodate shorter 10-cm or 20-cm needles for implanting superficial or deep-seated tumors.

Sterilization. The entire stainless steel tray and its contents may be sterilized by autoclaving just prior to use. The wooden case is used for transportation and shelf storage only.

Maintenance/cleaning. Immediately after the implant procedure and before commencement of the cleaning operations, all guide needles should be checked for possible remaining seeds. This check can be accomplished by inserting a wire through each needle. The instrument can be cleaned by soaking it in hydrogen peroxide immediately after use, followed by gentle scrubbing with a soft brush and spraying with jets of water. The sterilization tray can be cleaned with a regular stainless-steel cleaning spray. Use of an ultrasound cleaner is also recommended. When all parts are correctly stored it is immediately apparent if the set is complete (**Fig. 2-4**).

We have used the Mick applicator for more than a decade. In our experience it is reliable and relatively easy to use. It is important, however, that the operator not use excessive force on the stylet in the event of a stuck or locked I-125 seed to avoid damaging and possibly rupturing the seed.

IODINE-125 SEEDS IN CARRIERS (SUTURE SEEDS)

The term *seeds in carrier* refers to a group of 10 I-125 seeds within a mesh tube of Vicryl (polyglactin 910) absorbable suture material (**Fig. 2-5**). The seeds are spaced 1 cm apart, center to center. This ribbon is housed in a stainless-steel ring that provides complete shielding. The loaded ring is furnished in a ready-to-use sterile package (Medical-Surgical Division/3M, St Paul, MN).

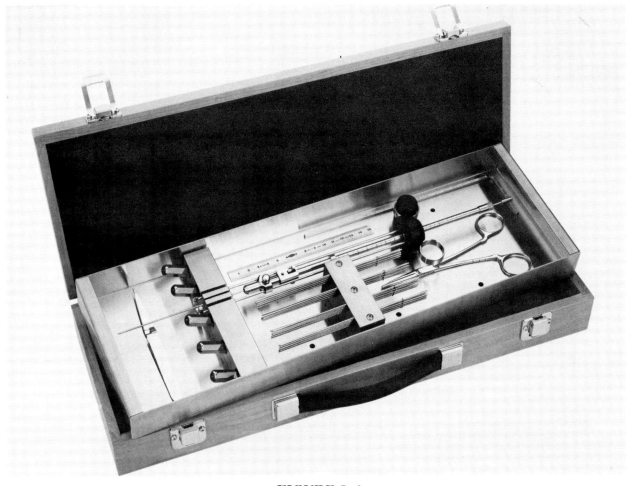

FIGURE 2-4

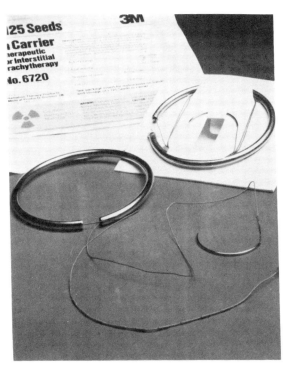

FIGURE 2-5

Temporary Implantation

The Ir-192 afterloading set used for temporary implantation should contain (**Fig. 2-6** and **Fig. 2-7**).

Straight stainless-steel needles, 17-cm gauge and 15-cm long.
Curved stainless-steel needles 15- and 20-cm long.
Nylon catheters 50-cm long with a thin leader portion.
Nylon catheters 50-cm long with a sealed end.
Stainless-steel buttons and/or plastic buttons, 1-cm diameter.
Plastic hemispherical spacers, 1-cm diameter, preferably transparent to separate the steel retainer buttons from the patient's skin.
15-cm stainless-steel rule.
Other equipment useful in certain techniques may be added, depending on the personal preference of the brachytherapist.

One standard afterloading set might be kept in the operating room, wrapped and sterile, so that an afterloading implant can be carried out without delay whenever an unresectable tumor is encountered. The set can be gas sterilized prior to its use. Autoclaving is not recommended because the plastic material used in the set can be damaged.

Iridium-192 in Plastic Ribbons

A plastic ribbon loaded with Ir-192 seeds, spaced 1 cm apart, is commercially available (Best Industries, Inc., Springfield, VA). The radioactive seeds are stainless-steel cylinders approximately 3 mm in length and 0.5 mm in diameter. A number of these ribbons are placed in a lead container, which is used for shipment, storage, and disposal of the radioactive seeds after their use. The lead container is placed in a bag for shipment and storage. For additional protection during shipment the lead container is placed in a wooden box with a lid secured by a seal. The seal is broken by the user and replaced with a padlock. For return shipment another seal, which is enclosed in the box, can be applied to the lid. No special tools are required.

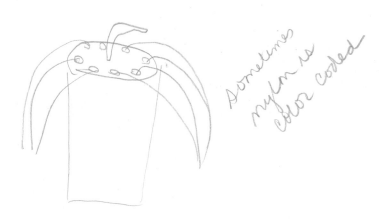

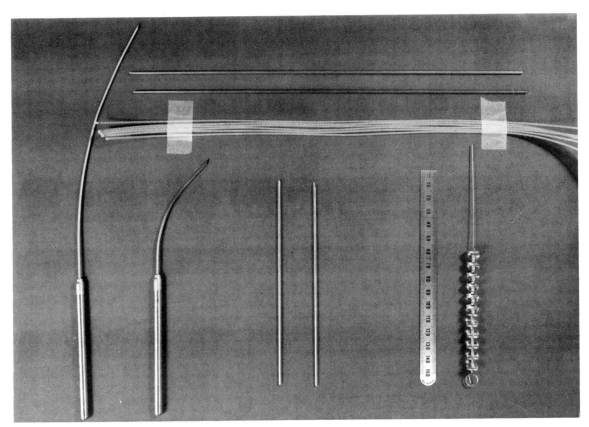

FIGURE 2-6

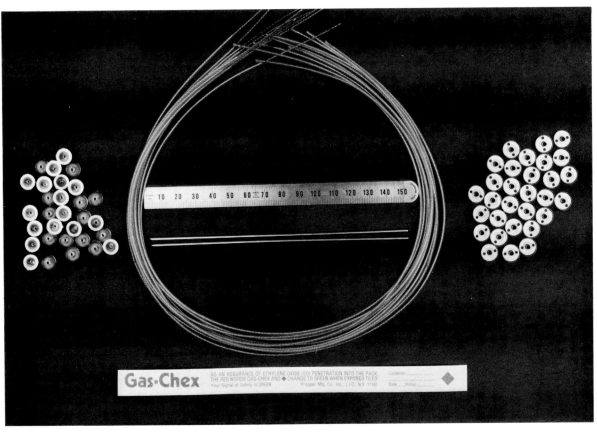

FIGURE 2-7

Stabilizers—Templates. Used to improve the accuracy of needle placement and to maintain needle position during treatment. Stabilizers are conveniently made of acrylic plastic and can be produced locally. Several designs are commercially available:

Syed-Neblett Gynecological Applicator (1). (**Fig. 2-8**). It consists of a perineal template, vaginal obturator, and a set of hollow needle source guides. The perineal template consists of two identical acrylic plates, each about 1-cm thick, superimposed and held together by six Allen-head screws. Both plates are drilled in an identical pattern to accept the guide needles. The vaginal obturator, 2-cm diameter and 15-cm long, has six grooves on its surface for the placement of guide needles and is centrally bored and threaded to accept an intrauterine tandem. The source guides for the Syed-Neblett applicator are 17-gauge hollow needles, 20-cm long, with blunt conical tips. All except the first guide have small metal rings near the distal end to prevent them from sliding proximally through the template. Recently, a disposable model of this applicator has become available.

Memorial Hospital Perineal Templates. These are customized templates used at Memorial Hospital mainly for perineal rectal (**Fig. 2-9**), prostate and/or gynecological implants (**Fig. 2-10**). Needle entry locations are selected to permit a match between the treatment-level isodose contour and a target region defined on computerized tomography (CT) scans.

Memorial Hospital Urethral Applicator (2). (**Fig. 2-11**). This applicator has been used by us for almost 20 years. This applicator consists of a template that permits the insertion of six needles in a circle around the urethra with a radius of 1 cm. The acrylic plastic template has a central hole through which a 28-gauge Foley catheter with a 30-cc bag is passed; a stainless-steel tube has been inserted into the rubber catheter for stabilization.

INTRACAVITARY BRACHYTHERAPY INSTRUMENTS

Intracavitary applicators have been used for the treatment of gynecological cancers for more than 50 years. Several applicators of many designs have been described and used. The most significant milestone in the evolution of applicator design was the introduction by Henschke of the afterloading principle, which has been adopted and incorporated in all currently used applicators.

FIGURE 2-8

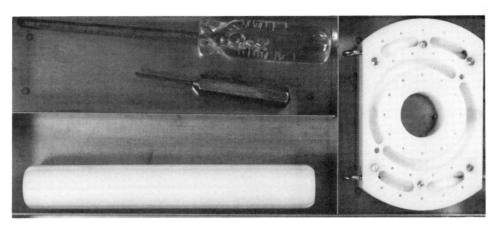

FIGURE 2-9

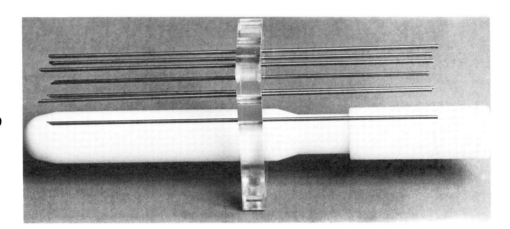

FIGURE 2-10

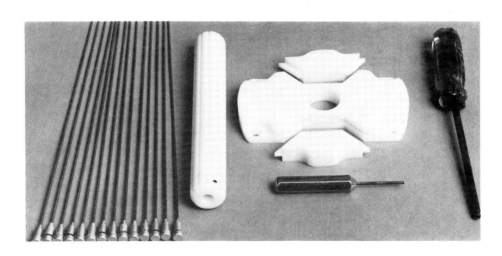

FIGURE 2-11

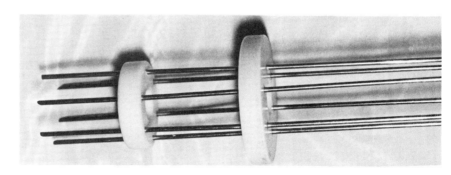

Henschke Afterloading Cervix Applicator (3,4) (Fig. 2-12).

Constructed mainly of stainless-steel, this applicator consists of a central uterine tube and two lateral vaginal tubes attached to one another by an adjustable-pivot yoke. Each lateral tube terminates in a hemispherical spacing colpostat of nylon. The applicator can be adapted to different anatomical conditions. To facilitate afterloading, new stainless-steel source carriers have been designed, with a spring-loaded end spacer that holds any number of sources securely in place. The intrauterine tube (tandem) is available in three different curvatures, with a cervical flange that can be moved to correspond to the length of the uterine cavity.

For each colpostat the smallest diameter (2 cm) ovoid is machined to accept anterior and posterior tungsten inserts for partial shielding of the bladder and rectum. These inserts are removable and can be replaced with nylon inserts as an option instead of the tungsten shield. Ovoid diameters of 2.5 cm (most often used) and 3 cm are achieved by adding hemospherical nylon caps. The stainless-steel yoke also serves to prevent dislocation or rotation of the uterine tube, which is fixed in the yoke by a knuckled set-screw that fits into a groove located on top of the uterine tube. Other adjustments are made by a single Allen wrench. Threaded end-caps are provided to cover each afterloaded tube (Fig. 2-13).

The applicator and its accessories can be either gas sterilized or autoclaved. For best cleaning results ultrasonic cleaning is recommended.

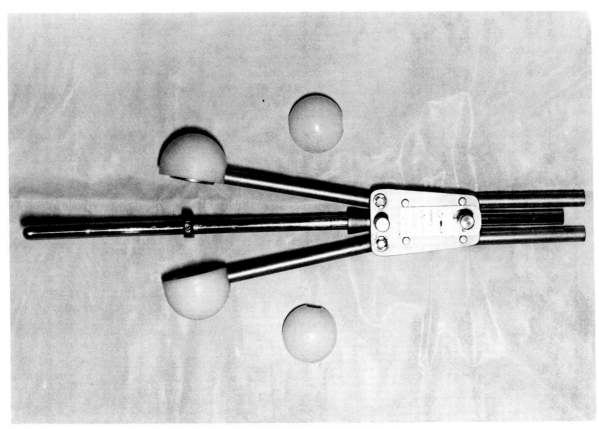

FIGURE 2-12

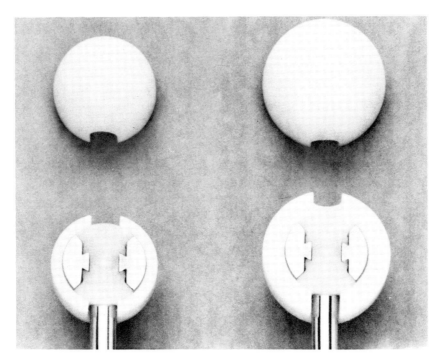

FIGURE 2-13

Fletcher Afterloading Cervix Applicator (5,6,7)

For which a recent commercially available version is the Fletcher–Suit–Delclos applicator (**Fig. 2-14**). This applicator is designed to have the vaginal source plane perpendicular to the vaginal axis, with medial tungsten shields at each end of cylindrical colpostats in order to reduce dose to the bladder and rectum. From left to right, this figure shows the standard applicator with afterloading colpostats (2 cm in diameter), plastic jackets used to increase the size to medium (2.5 cm in diameter) and large (3 cm in diameter), one applicator with half-cylinder colpostats (0.8 cm in radius) for narrow vaults (diameter when separated by the afterloading tandem is 3 cm), an assortment of three tandem tubes of the most useful curvatures with a metal flange having a "keel" to stabilize the tube in relation to packing placed around it (the flange is not needed if the tandem is used with vaginal cylinders), vaginal cylinders of different diameters and length to be used for the irradiation of selected regions of the vagina, inserters for the colpostats, and Teflon tubing to contain sources for insertion in the tandem.

Simon Capsules for Endometrial Cancer (8)

A uterine packing technique originally developed by Heyman to be used with radium capsules (**Fig. 2-15,** top), has been modified by Simon, who introduced an afterloading technique that uses a long plastic catheter with a nylon afterloading capsule at its tip (Fig. 2-15, bottom). Thin Cs-137 sources affixed to steel wires are afterloaded following the packing procedure. Beyond the lower radiation exposure associated with afterloading, the use of Simon's capsules has the further advantage of permitting meaningful dose calculations because inserted dummy sources can be individually localized radiographically.

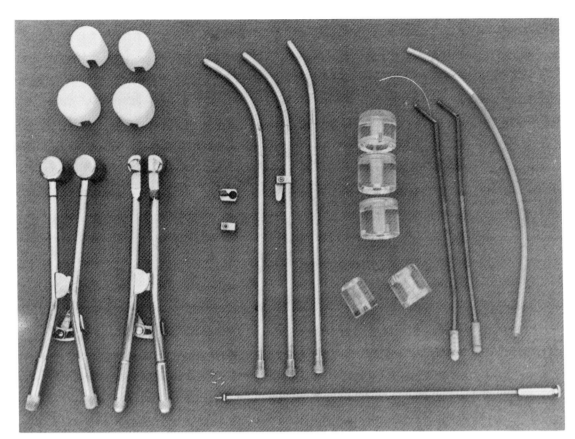

FIGURE 2-14

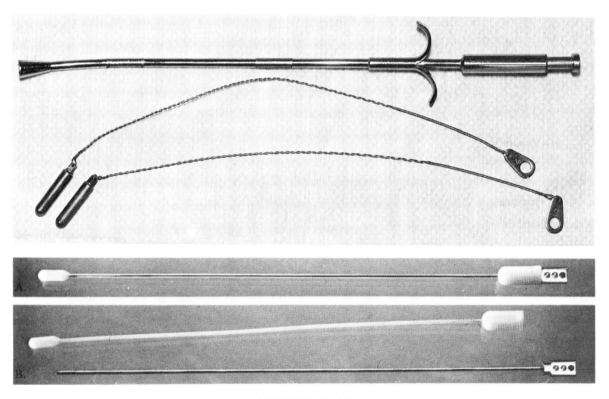

FIGURE 2-15

Hilaris–Nori Afterloading Endometrial Applicator (9) (Fig. 2-16)

An alternative to the packing technique, this applicator allows a wide range of adjustments of the dose distribution and permits irradiating both the uterus and the vagina in one step.

Each curved lateral tube is inserted into one of the cornua of the uterus with the straight tube placed in the center to improve the dose distribution in the fundus. All three tubes are fixed centrally in the vaginal cylinder, which is placed against the cervix. The vaginal cylinders supplied by the manufacturer vary in diameter (2.5 cm and 3 cm) and in length (6 to 12 cm). Radiopaque markers are located at the distal end of the vaginal cylinders, and a stainless-steel ring identifies the diameter and the length of the vaginal cylinder in use when radiographed.

One spacer tube is provided if only two tandems are inserted. Two locking devices, 2.5 cm and 3 cm, are supplied. Both locks snap into the marginal end of the vaginal cylinder. No screws or wrenches are needed. A lever protruding from the lock when pressed down firmly holds the tandems together.

Special Vaginal Applicators (Fig. 2-17)

These are special customized cylindrical vaginal applicators of various lengths and diameters designed to irradiate the whole vagina or the vaginal cuff in patients who have had a hysterectomy. Commercially produced vaginal applicators are also available.

REMOTE AFTERLOADING UNITS

Remote afterloading, which essentially eliminates staff exposure, was developed along two different lines. High dose rate remote afterloading is performed in a fully shielded facility; it permits treatment on an outpatient basis, by virtue of the short treatment time, but requires greater fractionation and reduction in total dose to achieve results comparable to low dose rate intracavitary brachytherapy. Low dose rate remote afterloading, on the other hand, utilizes conventional treatment times, enabling physicians to reproduce present treatment regimens. Although treatments are performed in the patient's hospital room, sources are retracted into a shielded position when staff or visitors enter. Supervision of afterloading machine operation requires technical personnel familiar with radiotherapeutic procedures who are able to handle possible emergency situations.

Remote afterloading varies widely in the extent to which custom optimization of dose distribution is feasible, i.e., in the extent to which the source configuration is readily adjustable.

Table 2-1 lists several remote afterloaders that have been distributed commercially, together with radionuclides used and modes of configuring and controlling sources for treatment. The table includes references to articles describing the development of these machines. Two widely used remote afterloaders with which the authors are familiar are the Gamma Med and the Selectron.

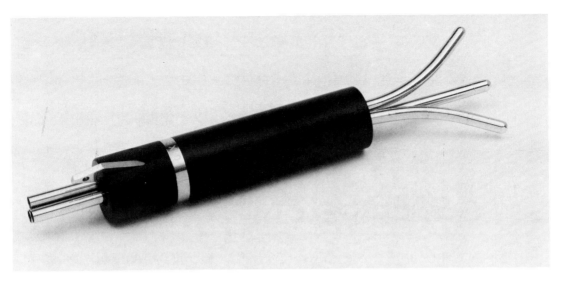

FIGURE 2-16

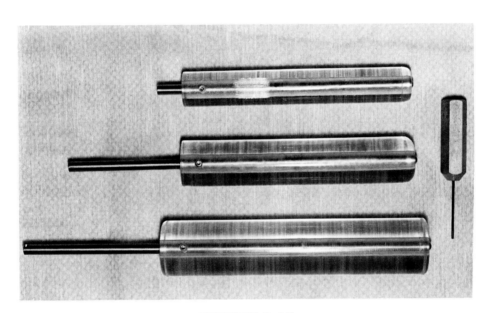

FIGURE 2-17

TABLE 2-1

Apparatus	Company	Radio Nuclides	Number Channels	Treatment Mode	References
Brachytron	AECL	Co-60	3	Oscillation	10,11
Buchler	Buchler	Ir-192 Cs-137	1	Oscillation	12
Cathetron	TEM	Co-60	3	Fixed preloaded	13,14
Cervitron II	Nuclesa	Cs-137	6	Fixed programmable	15
Curietron	CGR AGS	Cs-137 Ir-192	6	Fixed preloaded	16
Gamma Med II	Isotopen Technik	Ir-192	1	Stepping programmable	17,18
Ralstron	Shimadzu	Co-60	6	Fixed preloaded	19
Selectron	Nucletron	Cs-137 Ir-192	6	Fixed programmable	20

The Gamma-Med Remote Afterloader (Isotopen Technik, Haan, West Germany)

Employs a small Ir-192 source of nominally 370 GBq (10 Ci) and incorporates stepping-motor control of source position. With this unit, a single cable-mounted source may be positioned sequentially at each of 20 locations spaced uniformly (at a specified increment) within treatment catheters. Individual dwell times (in seconds) are specified, via a console keyboard, on the assumption of a 10-Ci source activity; actual dwell times are corrected automatically for decay, using the treatment-date entry, by an internal microprocessor. For high dose rate interstitial applications, the Gamma Med IIi incorporates an indexer (Mick Radio-Nuclear Instruments, Inc. Bronx, NY) to allow automatic switching of the source cable among implanted catheters (**Fig. 2-18**). Also available is a three-channel version (Gamma Med III) for low dose rate cervix applications using Cs-137 sources.

The Selectron Remote Afterloader (Nucletron Trading B.V., Leeersum, The Netherlands)

Was originally developed to achieve either low, medium, or high dose rates using small (2.5-mm diameter) spherical sources of different radionuclides (Cs-137, Ir-192, or Co-60) and various strengths. Sources are pneumatically driven into as many as six applicator catheters and are interspersed with inactive spheres of the same diameter in sequences that are separately programmable for each source train of 48 pellets. The Cs-137 unit for low and medium dose rates (**Fig. 2-19**) can be used to deliver intracavitary treatments for cervix cancer to two patients simultaneously. Subsequent developments have led to "micro" Selectron units: (1) a low and medium dose rate interstitial system using preloaded ribbons of either Ir-192 or Cs-137 seeds, and (2) a high dose rate interstitial and intraluminal system with stepping-motor control (in and among multiple catheters) of a small, cable-mounted Ir-192 source.

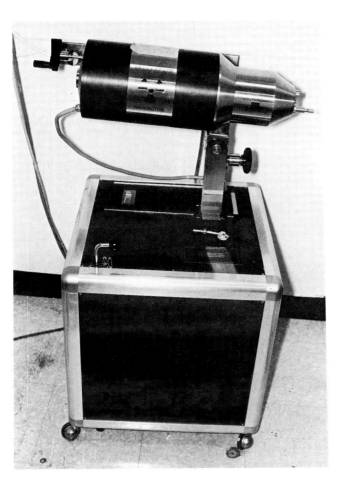

FIGURE 2-18

FIGURE 2-19

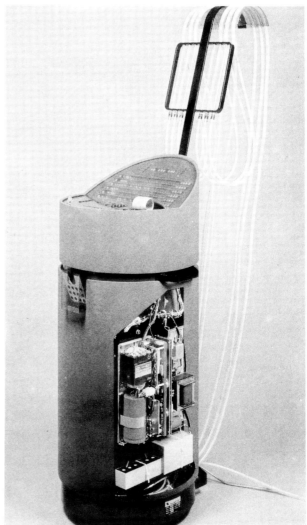

REFERENCES

1. D. Nori, B. Hilaris, (eds), Syed, A. M., and Puthawala, A. A. Interstitial-intracavitary "Syed–Neblett" applicator in the treatment of carcinoma of the cervix. In: *Radiation Therapy of Gynecological Cancer*. New York: Alan R. Liss, 1987, pp. 297–307.

2. Henschke, U. K., Hilaris, B. S., and Mahan, G. D. Afterloading in interstitial and intracavitary radiation therapy. *Am J Roentgenol Radium Ther and Nuclear Med* 90:386–395, 1963.

3. Henschke, U. K., Afterloading applicator for radiation therapy of carcinoma of uterus. *Radiology* 74:834, 1960.

4. Anderson, L. L., Masterson, M.E., and Nori, D. Intracavitary radiation treatment planning and dose evaluation. In: *Radiation Therapy of Gynecological Cancer*. New York: Alan R. Liss, 1987, pp. 51–71.

5. Fletcher, G. H., Shalek, R. J., Wall, J. A., and Bloedorn, F. G. A physical approach to the design of applicators in radium therapy of carcinoma of the cervix. *Am J Roentgenol* 68:935, 1952.

6. Suit, H. D., Moore, E. B., Fletcher G. H., and Worsnop, R. Modification of Fletcher ovoid system for afterloading using standard sized radium tubes (milligram and microgram). *Radiology* 81:126, 1963.

7. Delclos, L., Fletcher, G. H., Moore, E. B., and Sampiere, V. A. Minicolpostats, dome cylinders, other additions and improvements of the Fletcher-Suit afterloadable system: indications and limitations of their use. *Int J Radiat Oncol Biol Phys* 6:1195–1206, 1980.

8. Simon, N., and Silverstone, S. M. Intracavitary radiotherapy of endometrial cancer by afterloading. *Gynecol Oncol* 1:13–16, 1972.

9. Nori, D., Hilaris, B. S., and Anderson, L. A new endometrial applicator. *Int J Radiat Oncol Biol Phys* 8:941–945, 1982.

10. Henschke, U. K., Hilaris, B. S., and Mahan, G. D. Remote afterloading with intracavitary applicators. *Radiology* 83:344–345, 1964.

11. Von Essen, C. F., Seay, D. G., Moeller, M.S., and Hilbert, J. W. Fractionated intracavitary radiation therapy with the brachytron: general techniques and preliminary results in the treatment of cervix cancer. *Am J Roentgenol* 120:101–110, 1974.

12. Rotte, K., Linka, F., and Felder, K. D. Intrakavitare Bestrahlung des Uterus-karzinoms durch ein afterloading-gerat mit punkt-Iridium-192-quelle. *Strahlentherapie* 145:523–528, 1973.

13. O'Connell, D., Howard, N., Josling, C. A. F., Ramsey, N. W., and Liversage, W. E. A remotely controlled unit for the treatment of uterine carcinoma. *Lancet* 2:570, 1965.

14. O'Connell, D., Josling, C. A. F., Howard, N., Ramsey, N. W., and Liversage, W. E. The treatment of uterine carcinoma using the cathetron. Part I. Technique. *Br J Radiol* 40:882–887, 1967.

15. Cardis, R., and Kjellman, I. A new apparatus for intracavitary radiotherapy-cervitron II. In: Proc 5th Nordic Meeting on Clinical Physics, Stockholm, 1968.

16. Chassagne, D., DeLouche, G., Rocoplan, J. A., Pierquin, B., and Gest, J. Description et premiers essais due Curietron. *J Radiol Electrol* 50:910–913, 1969.

17. Mundinger, F., and Sauerwein, K. Gamma med, ein Gerat zur Bestrahlung von Hirngeschwulsten mit Radioisotopen. *Acta Radiol* 5:48–52, 1966.

18. Busch, M., Makosi, B., Schulz, U., and Sauerwein, K. Das Essener Nachlade-Verfahren fur die intrakavitare Strahlentherapie. *Strahlentherapie* 153:581–588, 1977.

19. Wakabayashi, M., Osawa, T., Mitsuhashi, H., Kikuchi, Y., Mita, M., Watanabe, T., Saito, K., Suda, Y., Yushii, M., Kato, S., Koshibu, R., Furuse, M., and Wakabayashi,

M. High dose rate intracavitary radiotherapy using the Ralstron. Introduction and Part I. (Treatment of carcinoma of the uterine cervix). *Nippon Acta Radiol* 31:340–378, 1971.

20. Van Hooft, E. The selectron. In: *Recent Advances in Brachytherapy Physics*, AAPM Monograph No. 7, Shearer, D. R. (ed.), New York: American Institute of Physics, 1981, pp. 167–177.

CHAPTER 3

Brachytherapy Techniques

INTERSTITIAL BRACHYTHERAPY

Interstitial brachytherapy is utilized today in the form of either temporary or permanent implants. In recent years, the number, complexity, and sophistication of brachytherapy techniques have markedly increased, attesting not only to the popularity of brachytherapy, but also to the ingenuity of radiation oncologists and scientists involved in this radiation subspecialty.

Modern Temporary Implant Techniques

Using either rigid needles or plastic flexible tubes these implants are currently afterloaded with Ir-192. These techniques will be discussed in detail as follows.

1. Basic temporary implant technique (1). Used for tumors that are readily accessible from opposite sides, as in the neck, breast, and skin. Both ends of the flexible plastic tubes lie outside the skin to which they are secured with metal buttons. Afterloading can thus be accomplished from either side. The principle steps in the basic technique are shown in **Fig. 3-1.** The first step is the insertion of a stainless-steel hypodermic needle (a). The second step is the threading of the leader (thin end) of the plastic tube through the stainless-steel needle until it emerges from the opposite end of the needle. The plastic leader and the needle are pulled through the tissue; the wider portion of the plastic tube follows behind the needle without trauma because this thicker portion of the tube has the same diameter as the needle (b). The third step is to attach the plastic hemisphere and the metal button to the protruding ends of the nylon tube and to secure the plastic tube on to the skin. This is accomplished by crimping the tubular part of the metal button with a hemostat, but only to the extent that it holds the plastic tube firmly in place without completely obstructing the lumen (c). The ends of the plastic tube are then cut off 3 to 4 cm beyond the metal button on each side. In a two- or more plane arrangement, the distance between planes and the distance of the superficial plane to the skin should be carefully measured with the help of a ruler (d).

To assure a good implant it is advisable to mark the needle position and the needle entrance and exit points on the patient's skin prior to insertion of the needles (**Fig. 3-2a**). Alignment of needles during the insertion is not

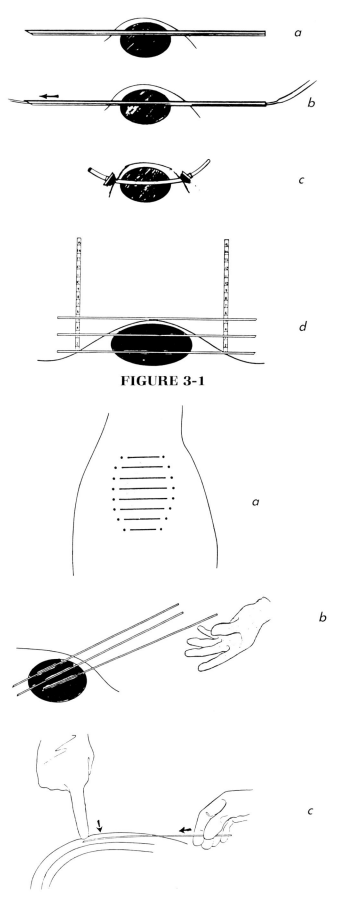

a

b

c

d

FIGURE 3-1

a

b

c

FIGURE 3-2

always easily accomplished; it can be carried out satisfactorily by holding the needle at its distal end and pushing it gently into the tissue (b). If the needle is not properly aligned, it should be removed and tried again. Implanting a curved surface with a straight needle is difficult and requires considerable skill. We have found that the placement of the needle is facilitated by palpating the needle tip with the index finger and guiding it slowly until the curvature is negotiated (c).

2. Loop implant technique (2,3,4,5). Used for the treatment of intraoral tumors, especially carcinoma of the tonsil, tongue, and floor of the mouth (**Fig. 3-3**). The loop implantation technique consists of the following steps:

1. A stainless-steel needle is inserted through the skin into the tumor and beyond it until the tip is felt by the finger. A second needle is introduced parallel to the first one in a similar way. The distance between the needles of the pair is 1 to 2 cm. The leader (thin end) of the afterloading plastic catheter is threaded through one of the needles and is pulled through the tumor into the oral cavity together with the needle.
2. The leader is now looped and threaded through the second needle of the pair; the leader and the needle are pulled slowly out of the tumor first, and then the skin, until the wider portion of the catheter becomes visible.
3. The outer ends of the nylon catheter are fixed on the skin, as in the basic temporary implant technique, with a plastic hemisphere and a metal button.

A modification of the loop technique is shown in **Fig. 3-4.** This technique is useful for tumors that are in the oropharynx, such as on the base of the tongue, and are not easily visualized.

1. Following the insertion of a pair of needles, as in the previous technique, a thin wire loop is threaded through the first needle, and the needle is removed
2. The thin end of the nylon catheter is threaded through the wire loop; the wire is pulled, first bringing the thin end, and then the wide portion of the catheter, into the mouth.
3. The wire loop is now threaded through the second needle. The needle, wire, and part of the nylon catheter are pulled out of the mouth.
4. Finally, both ends of the nylon catheter are secured on the skin.

The separation between the arms of the loop is 1.2 to 1.5 cm, with the larger separation used for larger tumors. The peripheral catheters should be 0.5 cm beyond the tumor margin.

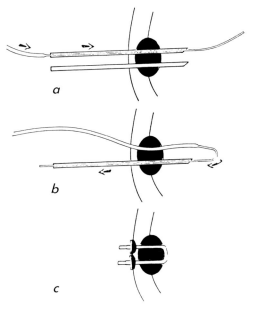

FIGURE 3-3

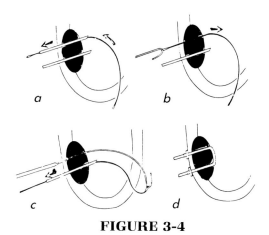

FIGURE 3-4

3. Guide gutter technique (6).   This is a further modification of the loop technique, popularized by Pierquin in France. This technique is useful in the management of intraoral lesions, especially small tumors of the mobile portion of the tongue, floor of the mouth, and tonsil. It was developed to be used with Ir-192 wires.

Figure 3-5 shows a double guide gutter.

1. The length of each arm of the double gutter is 3.5 cm and the separation between the pins is 1.2 cm. Each pin has a medial slit to allow the subsequent removal of the gutter after the afterloading of the Ir-192 wires.
2. The Ir-192 wire used for the afterloading of a double guide gutter resembles a hairpin.
3. The radioactive Ir-192 hairpin is held with a forcep and introduced simultaneously into both arms of the double gutter.
4. To remove the guide gutter after the insertion of the hairpin, a long forcep is placed over the transverse section of the radioactive hairpin to hold it down on the surface of the tissue, while with another forcep the guide gutter is slowly removed from the tissue, leaving the hairpin in place. To prevent slippage the hairpin is tied on the mucosa with a silk tie.

4. Sealed-end technique (7).   Utilized in tumors accessible from only one side, usually in the thoracic, abdominal, and pelvic cavities. The one end of the plastic tube is sealed to avoid communication with the outside and therefore prevent infection (**Fig. 3-6**).

1. A 17-gauge hypodermic needle is inserted through the skin into the tumor.
2. The sealed end of the plastic tube is inserted in the needle and pushed in until it reaches the tip of the needle.
3. The needle is withdrawn and the tube is secured on the skin with a plastic hemisphere and a metal button. To secure the plastic tube from slipping, a silk suture is threaded through each one of the button's holes and sutured on the skin.

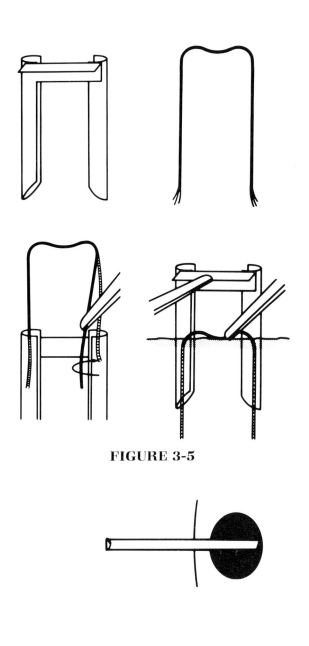

FIGURE 3-5

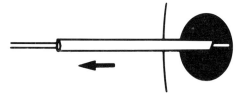

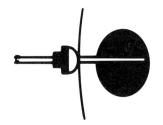

FIGURE 3-6

5. Suture technique (2). This is helpful in the treatment of intraabdominal tumors, especially bladder carcinoma (**Fig. 3-7**).

1. The thin end (leader) of a plastic catheter is threaded through the eye of a surgical needle—usually the largest curved needle available in the operating room. This curved needle is sutured through the bladder wall about 2 cm superior to the tumor; it is pushed through the bladder wall at the base of the tumor and exists about 2 cm inferior to the tumor.
2. The wide part of the nylon catheter is inserted into the bladder wall; while the curved needle with the leader is brought out through the skin.
3. The tube is secured on the anterior abdominal wall, lateral to the surgical incision, in the usual manner with a plastic hemisphere and a metal button; and the leader is cut off 3 to 4 cm from its exit point. The metal button is fastened on the skin with a silk suture that is threaded through each one of the two button holes.
4. The same steps are repeated until the entire tumor is covered with the appropriate number of plastic catheters. The separation of the catheters is determined by the use of the appropriate nomogram (see Chap. 4).

6. Tumor bed implant technique. This is used when the initial management of a cancerous lesion is by surgical resection, especially when it is suspected that the surgical margin is not adequate. Either the temporary basic or sealed-end technique or the permanent gelfoam technique can be used for this type of implant.

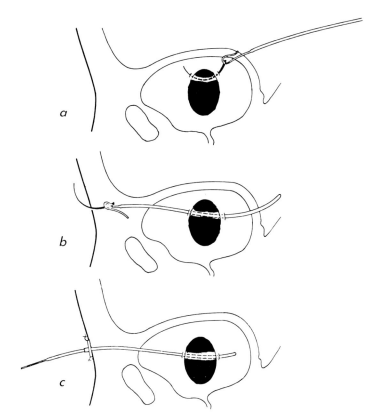

FIGURE 3-7

Afterloading with Iridium-192 in Plastic Ribbons.   The technique of after-loading the Ir-192 ribbons into the previously implanted plastic catheters (in the basic technique) is shown in **Fig. 3-8**. Before the afterloading is started, the number of seeds in each ribbon is recorded. In a complicated implant, it is a good practice to attach a small piece of tape with the desired number of seeds on each afterloading plastic catheter.

1. To reduce radiation exposure, all ribbon leaders are first threaded through each plastic catheter, before any active sources are pulled into position.
2. Using a long forcep, the source-containing end of the nylon ribbon is pulled out of the lead container and the radioactive sources that are not needed are cut off.
3. The nylon ribbon is pulled into the plastic catheter as far as indicated (allowing at least a 0.5-cm clearance between each end-seed and skin) and is secured in position by crimping the tubular portion of the metal button with a heavy clamp. The nylon ribbon can be cut 1 to 2 cm beyond its exit from the plastic catheter or left in the original length if reuse is planned.

Blind end

This process is repeated with the remaining plastic tubes until all of them have been afterloaded. If the suture or the sealed-end technique has been used for the implantation of the plastic catheters, the portion of each ribbon containing the radioactive sources must be inserted first. This modified loading technique results in a somewhat higher radiation exposure to the operator, unless he or she works behind a lead screen. The threading of the active portion of the Ir-192 containing nylon ribbon into the plastic catheter may be facilitated by using a funnel placed over the outer plastic tube to guide the nylon ribbon.

Removal and Disposal of Iridium-192 Seeds.   To reduce radiation exposure it is essential to remove the nylon ribbons with the Ir-192 seeds as quickly as possible. This is accomplished by means of a commercially available special instrument that resembles an electrical wire stripper and which cuts only the outer plastic tube, not the inner nylon ribbon. Its use is illustrated in **Fig. 3-9**. The instrument is applied directly in front of the metal button and is closed (a). This movement cuts the outer tube while gripping the nylon ribbon firmly enough so that it can be removed in the same motion.

A Geiger counter or other sensitive rate meter should always be on hand during the removal of the sources. The patient, as well as the room, should be checked at the end of the removal to make certain that no Ir-192 seeds were lost. Instruments that are at least 20-cm long should be used in handling the active ends of the Ir-192 nylon ribbons.

The lead container holding the seeds is returned in the shipping box to the supplier for disposal. Thus, no special storage or disposal facilities are required with this technique.

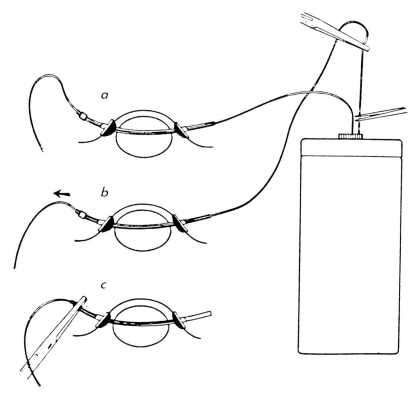

Afterloading of iridium-192 seeds in nylon ribbons.

FIGURE 3-8

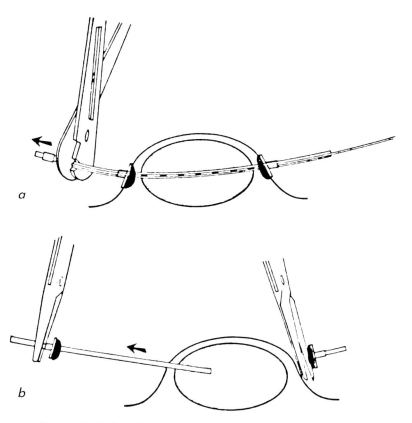

Removal of nylon ribbons.

FIGURE 3-9

Modern Permanent Implant Techniques

These utilize individual single seeds, seeds loaded in magazines, and seeds loaded into absorbable Vicryl sutures, which can be inserted into tumors percutaneously under local anesthesia or sedation as well as intraoperatively under general anesthesia.

1. Basic permanent implant technique (8). This is used in tumors in which a volume implant is required. Seed inserters, commonly with preloaded magazines, are commercially available to be used with this technique.

The first step of this permanent interstitial implant technique is shown on the left of **Fig. 3-10**. Hollow 17-gauge stainless-steel hypodermic needles, 15-cm long, tips ground with a 45-degree bevel, are inserted into the tumor. For implants through the intact skin, needles with sharper points are preferable, but for intrathoracic and intraabdominal implants it is better to have needles that do not penetrate the tissues as easily. In this way the tissue resistance, which is often crucial for defining the margins of a tumor, is more readily determined. Another advantage of using blunter needles is that they do not change their position in the tissue as easily as do the more sharply tapered ones.

The hollow needles are inserted around the periphery of the tumor mass first. If possible, all needles are inserted parallel to one another. The direction of the needles must be considered carefully before starting the procedure so that their position may be palpated and the maximum number of seeds may be inserted through one needle. The number of needles and their spacing is determined by an appropriate nomogram (see New York System of dosimetry in Chap. 4).

The second step of this technique, shown on the right of this figure, is the afterloading of the needles with the radioactive seeds using a commercially available source inserter.

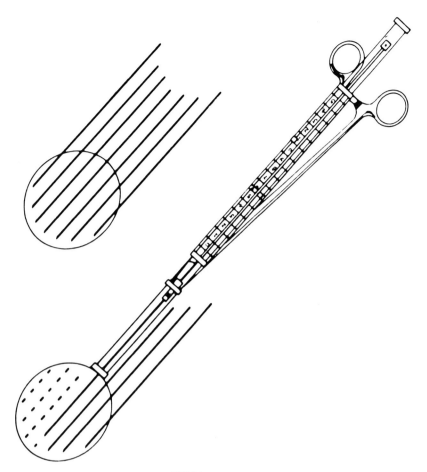

FIGURE 3-10

2. Absorbable Vicryl suture technique (9,10). This is useful for planar implants in head and neck, chest wall, and pelvic side wall tumors, when single seeds cannot be used, either because of tumor necrosis or inadequate tissue. I-125 seeds loaded into absorbable Vicryl suture are commercially available. After the completion of the surgical resection, and the determination of the target dimensions, the vicryl sutures are sewn into the tissues, using the attached needle, with the precalculated spacing between each suture. The target region is measured in its length and width. The number of radioactive seeds necessary to give a peripheral dose of 16,000 cGy is estimated using a variation of the planar implant nomograph. After the I-125 seeds are pulled into position, Weck clips are attached at each end of the suture and the excess suture material is cut off, resulting in a regularly spaced planar implant. The wound is then closed, completing the procedure (**Fig. 3-11**).

3. Gelfoam-impregnated I-125 seed technique (11). This is a relatively more simple method to implant permanently small residual tumors when neither the basic permanent implant technique nor the absorbable Vicryl suture method are suitable because of an inadequate tissue stroma or the proximity of vulnerable structures.

After surgical resection, the tumor bed is demarcated by surgical clips. The target region is measured in its length and width and the number of radioactive seeds necessary to give a minimum peripheral dose of 16,000 cGy is estimated as before. An absorbable gelatin sponge (gelfoam) with the measured dimensions of the target region is prepared and the recommended position of the suture is marked on it (**Fig. 3-12,** left). The I-125 suture is sewn through the sponge with its ends clipped to keep the suture within the sponge (Fig. 3-12, right).

When seeds in suture are not available, loose I-125 seeds can be implanted in the gelfoam plaque. A matrix is drawn on the gelfoam with mesh points corresponding to where each seed should be placed (Fig. 3-13, left); the magazine containing the seeds is attached to a Mick applicator; and the needle is placed on the mesh point with the bevelled tip slightly below the surface of the gelfoam to allow space for the I-125 seeds. A seed is then expelled gently, the needle is withdrawn, and the process is repeated at the next mesh point until all of the points are covered. Next, a layer of sterile lubricant (surgilube) is applied to the surface of the gelfoam. At this point another piece of gelfoam of equal dimensions is "sandwiched" to the radioactive gelfoam plaque using large hemoclips (**Fig. 3-13,** right). This gelfoam sandwich can then be secured onto the tumor bed.

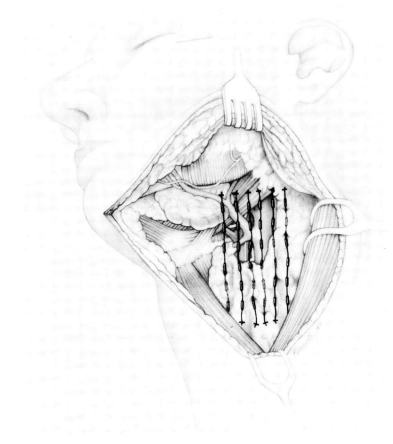

FIGURE 3-11

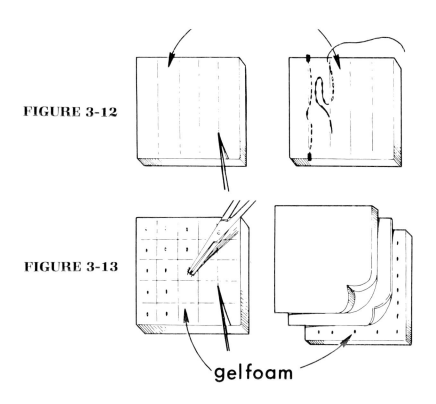

FIGURE 3-12

FIGURE 3-13

gelfoam

Special Interstitial Techniques

1. Stabilizer (template) techniques. These are used in the treatment of accessible tumors. In our experience accessibility is most frequently associated with the perineum, vagina, female urethra, and chest wall. The templates are usually made of acrylic plastic and are secured to the skin by silk suture or adhesive tape to prevent slippage of the stainless-steel needles. These templates are commercially available or custom made (**Fig. 3-14**). The main advantages of template techniques are the improved accuracy of placement of radioactive sources, the easy reproducibility of the brachytherapy technique, and the proper maintenance of source position during treatment. Templates allow the newcomer in brachytherapy to achieve in some situations what ordinarily would have required several years of training and experience. Specific applications of templates will be discussed in subsequent chapters.

2. Stereotactic techniques (12,13,14,15,16). These are used for deep-seated tumors, such as brain, prostate, pancreas, and peripheral lung, and are assisted by CT or sonography. Dose optimization programs to find the best source location, with computer-controlled positioning devices to implement them have a great potential.

Figure 3-15 shows the type of stereotactic device employed for brain implants. This stereotactic frame is applied under local anesthesia, usually the day before the implantation, to allow the performance of a CT scan for implant planning. Details of its clinical application will be discussed in another chapter (brain).

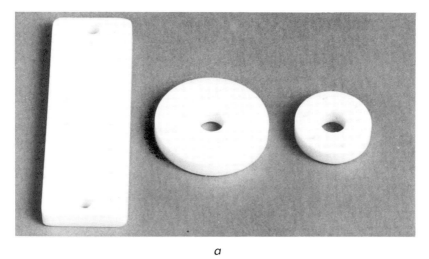

a

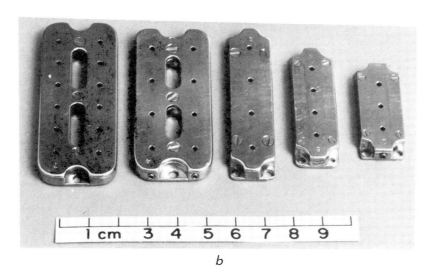

b

FIGURE 3-14

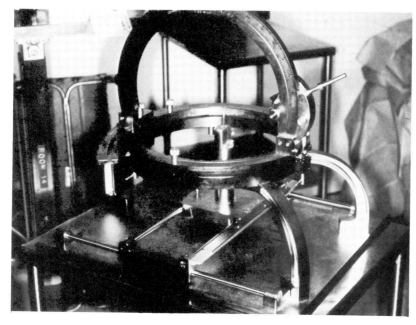

FIGURE 3-15

3. Eye plaque techniques (17,18). These are used today with I-125 rather than Co-60 because of the ease of shielding and the resulting negligible radiation to the extraorbital tissues. Eye plaques have been used to treat intraocular posterior segment tumors, mainly choroidal melanoma, in an attempt to avoid enucleation and preserve a functioning eye. More recently, an eye plaque has been developed that incorporates a microwave antenna in addition to I-125 seeds, permitting hyperthermia and brachytherapy to be applied simultaneously. The dimensions of the tumor are obtained from fundus examination and from ultrasound, usually with 1- to 2-mm margin all around.

Computer planning programs are used to optimize the seed number and arrangement for I-125 plaques. The I-125 seeds are sandwiched between a gold outer plaque and an inner plastic plaque. The gold outer plaque has a lip or edge shield that encircles the plaque and extends to the sclera. The activity and number of seeds is chosen so that the dose rate at the prescription point at the apex of the tumor is between 50 and 125 cGy per hour. The plaques are provided with suture holes in at least two positions on the periphery of the plaque. The placement of the plaque is done intraoperatively (**Fig. 3-16**).

4. Mould techniques (19). These are currently of limited application. Moulds are prepared on an individual basis, usually of plastic material and varied according to the anatomic site. The number of radioactive seeds, their placement in relation to the surface of the mould, and their strength are predetermined. The sources are afterloaded either manually or remotely after the mould has been positioned under local anesthesia or sedation. Sources with low energy, such as I-125, have the advantage of easy shielding of the neighboring normal tissue (**Fig. 3-17**).

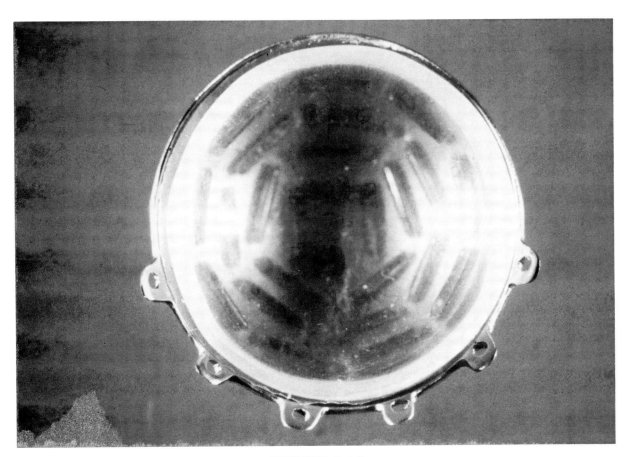

FIGURE 3-16

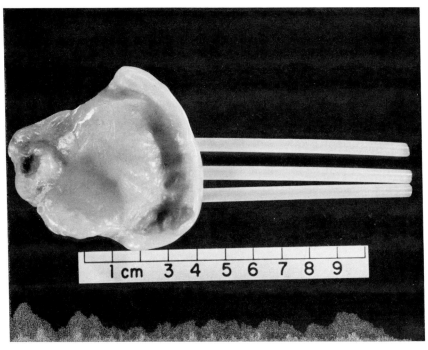

FIGURE 3-17

INTRACAVITARY BRACHYTHERAPY TECHNIQUES

Intracavitary brachytherapy has been a mainstay in the treatment of uterine cervix cancer for more than 50 years. In the course of this long history, applicators of a great many designs have been described and used. The most significant milestone in the evolution of applicator design was the introduction by Henschke of the afterloading principle, with its manifest radiation protection advantages. The main advantage of an intracavitary application is the ease of insertion. The main disadvantage is the relatively low depth dose because the fall-off of the dose is very rapid. The fall-off from the source is not as pronounced, however, if a long linear source is used instead of a point source; or if the distance between the source and the irradiated surface is increased. The most efficient method to increase the dose to the tumor, however, is by cross-firing it with two or more sources. This is the case in the treatment of cancer of the cervix by using a combination of intrauterine and intravaginal sources.

Modern intracavitary techniques for gynecologic and other sites have generally been designed for manual afterloading. While manual afterloading eliminates radiation exposure in the operating room and recovery room, radiation protection during the loading, transport, insertion, and removal of sources, and during the nursing care of the patient under treatment continues to be a major problem. In order to remedy this situation remote afterloading was developed that eliminates the radiation exposure completely.

Modern Manual Intracavitary Techniques

1. Cancer of the cervix technique (20).   **Figure 3-18** shows the afterloading technique for cancer of the cervix. The first step is the insertion of the unloaded applicator, which is usually performed under general anesthesia in the operating room. The second step is the afterloading with the radioactive sources, which is usually done after the patient has returned to her room and after localization x-rays have been taken and the dosimetry has been completed.

The Henschke applicator, in either the original or its improved version, has been in continuous use at Memorial Hospital since its introduction in 1960. Designed primarily to facilitate afterloading in cervix intracavitary brachytherapy, the Henschke applicator meets generally accepted requirements for versatility and durability. Its ovoid-type colpostat is advantageous with respect both to ease of insertion and dose uniformity. Its rigid construction assures reliable delivery of a tailored dose distribution as it is shown in these two radiographs taken in an anterioposterior and a lateral projection (**Fig. 3-19**). Its utility is enhanced by the addition to the colpostat of rectal and bladder shields.

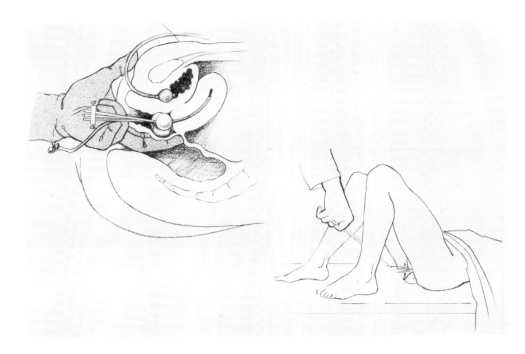

FIGURE 3-18

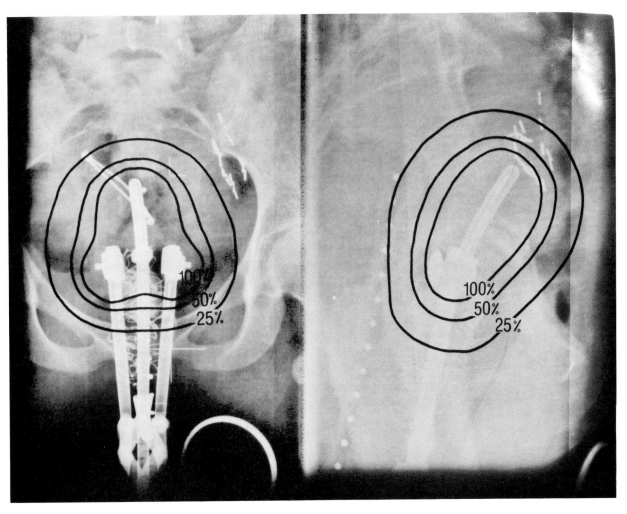

FIGURE 3-19

2. *Cancer of the corpus intracavitary techniques.* The original intrauterine packing technique of the uterine cavity was described by Heyman and utilized preloaded radium capsules. With the packing technique, a more homogeneous distribution of the radiation is achieved by stretching the uterine cavity than was achieved by a single uterine tandem. This technique has been modified by Simon, who used disposable Teflon® capsules afterloaded with small Cs-137 sources. In order to maintain the afterloading principle, utilized at Memorial Hospital in all interstitial and intracavitary techniques, we developed an applicator for the treatment of cancer of the corpus in 1967. **Figure 3-20** shows, from left to right, the applicator properly positioned within a hysterectomy specimen and the idealized alignment of the preoperatively calculated dose distribution within the actual specimen. It also shows the recommended source position, activity in milligram Radium equivalent, and dose distribution in anterioposterior and lateral projections. The applicator is loaded with Cs-137 sources for manual afterloading; however, high activity Co-60 or Ir-192 sources can be used for remote afterloading.

Remote Afterloading Techniques

1. *Low dose rate remote afterloading techniques.* Except for the programming and attachment of the machine controlling source movement, these techniques involve procedural steps identical to the ones described previously for manual afterloading.

2. *High dose rate remote afterloading techniques (21,22).* In addition to their obvious advantages of treatment on an outpatient basis, and their short treatment time, these techniques allow a controlled temporary displacement of normal structures during the brief treatment interval to achieve dose reductions that would not be possible with more protracted treatments. Such an intraoperative application, suitable for tumor bed irradiation (paraaortic nodes) is shown in **Fig. 3-21**. The achievable dose distribution in an anterioposterior projection (left), in a lateral (right upper), and in transverse (right lower) demonstrates the ability to deliver an intraoperative boost dose of 600 cGy to the paraaortic nodes while sparing the neighboring bowel. Intracavitary high dose rate techniques used in cancer of the cervix and corpus, as well as in other sites, i.e., trachea, esophagus, nasopharynx, rectum, and bladder, have gained wide appeal in the last few years. They will be discussed further in the subsequent chapters.

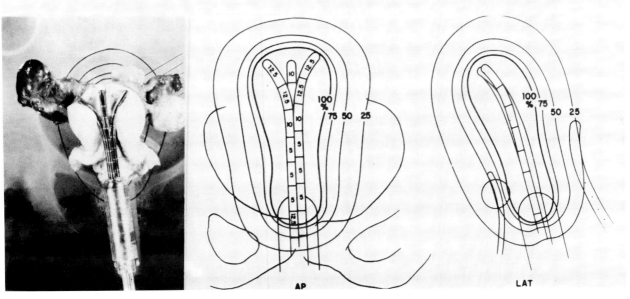

FIGURE 3-20

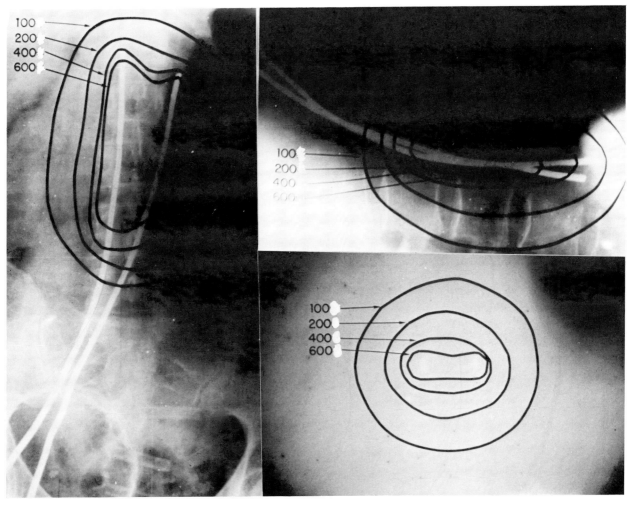

FIGURE 3-21

REFERENCES

1. Henschke, U. K., and Hilaris, B. S. Afterloading for interstitial gamma ray implantation. In: Fletcher G. H. (ed). *Textbook of Radiotherapy*. Philadelphia; Lea & Febiger, 1966, pp. 39–44.

2. Hilaris, B. S., and Henschke, U. K. General principles and techniques of interstitial brachytherapy. In: Hilaris, B. S. (ed). *Handbook of Interstitial Brachytherapy*. Acton, Mass.: Publishing Sciences Group, 1975, pp. 69–81.

3. Henschke, U. K., Cowan, L., Goldson, A., Hill, L., Hintz, B., Kumar, P., Mahan, D., Nibhanupudy, R., Syed, M., Suthanthiran, K., and Tabron, M. Potential and practice for head and neck implant. In: *Proceedings of the 13th International Congress of Radiology*, Madrid, 1973, Vol. 2:15–20. Amsterdam, *Excerpta Med*: 189–192, 1974.

4. Levine, W., Wasserman, H. J. An improved technique of interstitial radiotherapy of the tongue. *Br J Radiol* 51:213–217, 1978.

5. Vikram, B., and Hilaris, B. S. A non-looping afterloading technique for interstitial implants of the base of the tongue. *Int J Radiat Oncol Biol Phys* 7:419–422, 1981.

6. Pierquin, B., Chassagne, D., Issa, P., and Vandenbrouch, C. L'endocurietherapie des carcinomas epidermoides du voile par l'Iridium 192. *J Radiol* 50:23–27, 1969.

7. Hilaris, B. S., Nori, D., and Anderson, L. L. New approaches to brachytherapy. In: DeVita, V. T., Hellman, S., and Rosenberg, S.A. (eds.), *Important Advances in Oncology 1987*, Chapter 12, Part Two: Clinical Progress. 1987, Philadelphia: J. B. Lippincott Co., pp. 237–261.

8. Henschke, U. K. Technic for permanent implantation of radioisotopes. *Radiology* 68:256, 1957.

9. Martinez, A., Goffinet, D. R., Fee, W., Goode, R., Palos, B., Cox, R., and Pooler, D. ^{125}Iodine suture implants as an adjuvant to surgery and external beam radiotherapy in the management of locally advanced head and neck cancer. *Cancer* 51:973–979, 1983.

10. Goffinet, D. F., Martinez, A., and Fee, W. E., Jr. ^{125}I vicryl suture implants as a surgical adjuvant in cancer of the head and neck. *Int J Radiat Oncol Biol Phys* 11:399–402, 1985.

11. Marchese, M. J., Nori, D., Anderson, L. L., and Hilaris, B. S. A versatile permanent planar implant technique utilizing iodine-125 seeds imbedded in gelfoam. *Int J Radiat Oncol Biol Phys* 10:747–751, 1984.

12. Mundinger, F. Treatment of small cerebral gliomas with CT aided stereotactic curietherapy. *Neuroradiology* 16:564–567, 1978.

13. Rossman, K. J., Shetter, A. G., Speiser, B. L., and Nehls, D. Stereotactic afterloading iridium implants in treatment of high-grade astrocytomas. *Endocuriether Hyperthermia Oncol* 1:49–57, 1985.

14. Holm, H. H., Stroyer, I., Hansen, H., and Stadil, F. Ultrasonically guided percutaneous interstitial implantation of iodine-125 seeds in cancer therapy. *Br J Radiol* 54:665–670, 1981.

15. Holm, H. H., Juul, N., Pedersen, J. F., Hansen, H., and Stroyer, I. Transperineal iodine-125 seed implantation in prostatic cancer guided by transrectal ultrasonography. *J Urol* 130:282–286, 1983.

16. Nag, S. Transperineal iodine-125 implantation of the prostate under transrectal ultrasound and fluoroscopic control. *Endocuriether Hyperthermia Oncol* 1:207–212, 1985.

17. Robertson, D. M., Earle, J., and Anderson, J. A. Preliminary observations regarding the use of iodine-125 in the management of choroidal melanomas. *Trans Ophthalmol Soc UK* 103:155–160, 1983.

18. Rotman, M., Packer, S., Bosworth, J., and Chiu-Tsao, S. T. I-125 ophthalmic appli-

cators in the treatment of choroidal melanoma (abstr). *Int J Radiat Oncol Biol Phys* 10:107–108, 1984.

19. Bauer, M., Schultz-Wendtland, R., Fritz, P., and Winkel, K. Z. Contact therapy of tumor recurrences in the regions of the pharynx and oral cavity by means of remote-controlled afterloading technique. *Endocuriether Hyperthermia Oncol* 2:37–42, 1986.

20. Brown, S. G. Radiation therapy in the treatment of carcinoma of the cervix. Nori, D., and Hilaris, B. S. (eds.). In: *Radiation Therapy of Gynecological Cancer.* New York; Alan R. Liss, 1987, pp. 101–114.

21. Nori, D., Hilaris, B. S., Chadha, M., Bains, M., Jain, S., Hopfan, S., and Anderson, L. L. Clinical applications of a remote afterloader. *Endocuriether Hyperthermia Oncol* 1:193–200, 1985.

22. Henschke, U. K., Hilaris, B. S., and Mahan, G. D. Remote afterloading with intracavitary applicators. *Radiology* 83:344–345, 1964.

CHAPTER 4

Interstitial Brachytherapy Planning and Evaluation

INTERSTITIAL BRACHYTHERAPY

In the traditional approach to interstitial treatment planning, e.g., the Manchester system, the target region size (area or volume) is determined and a table or graph is consulted to determine the amount of radium required to deliver a desired peripheral dose. The radioactive sources are arranged according to certain "distribution rules" to produce uniform radiation over the treated area or within the treated volume. The advent of computers made it possible to generate large amounts of data quickly, and to accomplish planning by trying various source configurations until a satisfactory dose distribution was obtained. Subsequently, the focus was on methods of reducing the abundant computer data to manageable proportions, i.e., to a few, meaningful numbers in evaluation. Currently, the computer is increasingly being asked to evaluate intermediate dose distributions and to rearrange sources appropriately, as well as to assist in forming 3-D anatomical images for more accurate target definition.

Tumor and Target Volume

The tumor volume is determined by clinical, radiographic, computed tomography (CT), and exploratory operative examinations. Following the histological diagnosis of cancer, palpation may, in some instances, provide a good estimate of the size of the tumor and its extension into nearby normal tissues such as skin, nerves, vessels and bone. Appropriate imaging studies, e.g., radiography, CT (**Fig. 4-1**), nuclear scanning, ultrasound, and examination under anesthesia will enable the physician to define more precisely the tumor extent. In intrathoracic and intraabdominal cancer, however, the most valuable procedure is surgical exploration, with pathological examination of suspicious areas and placement of surgical clips to outline the tumor region.

Target volume includes the tumor volume and an adequate margin of normal tissue varying from 1 to 2 cm in the head and neck region (**Fig. 4-2**) to 4 to 5 cm in the extremities. It is the region within which the radiation dose is equal to or greater than the prescribed dose.

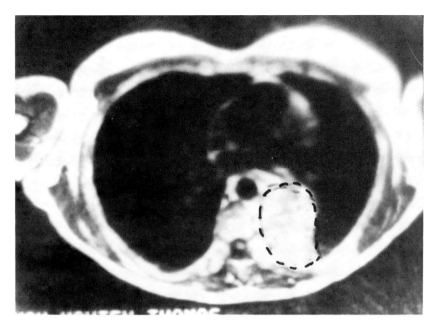

FIGURE 4-1

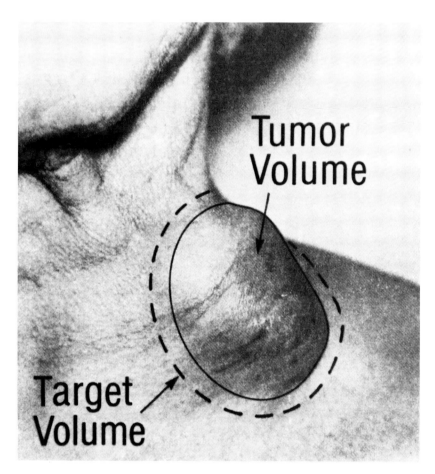

FIGURE 4-2

Selection of Type, Geometry of Implant, and Radionuclide

The decision whether a permanent or temporary implant is required, and the definition of the geometry of the implant, e.g., one-plane, two-plane, or volume, is based on the size, location, and spread of the tumor and on the proximity of normal structures. The latter concern may lead to a decision to use a low-energy radionuclide, such as I-125, for a temporary implant to limit dose to critical structures, i.e., spinal cord, eye, or gonads.

Techniques for the two types of interstitial brachytherapy, *temporary* and *permanent implants*, have already been discussed. Temporary implants are generally used in the treatment of cancers of the brain, head and neck region (lip, floor of the mouth, tongue, buccal mucosa, and nasopharynx), breast, soft tissue sarcoma of the extremities and trunk, bladder, vagina and vulva, urethra, and thoracic wall. Permanent implants are used in the brain, other head and neck sites, prostate, lung, pancreas, and gynecological sites.

There is considerable overlap between the indications for temporary and permanent implants. With skill and experience on the part of the physician and with the availability of special instruments and insertion techniques (templates, stereotactic devices), the same accuracy of source placement and dose distribution can be closely attained with permanent as well as with temporary implants. On the other hand, the inherent advantages of permitting adjustments of source distribution during treatment and of affording control over treatment time with temporary implants frequently makes the use of temporary implants preferable even in the thoracic or the abdominal cavity.

A *planar implant* is adequate for target regions less than 1.5-cm thick. Planning is usually based on a rectangular arrangement of uniformly spaced, parallel source lines (wires or ribbons). Single-plane implants (**Fig. 4-3**) are useful for treating either relatively flat lesions, spreading along surfaces such as the neck or the chest wall, or for surgical-fields following excision of the tumor. A *two-plane implant* (**Fig. 4-4**) is recommended for targets 1.5- to 2.5-cm thick. The spacing between source lines in each plane varies from 1 to 1.5 cm. A *volume implant* (**Fig. 4-5**) is suitable for targets involving larger tumors embedded in tissue that can be implanted throughout such as intrathoracic or intraabdominal tumors.

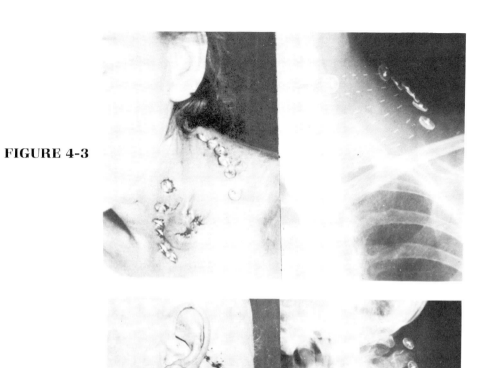

FIGURE 4-3

FIGURE 4-4

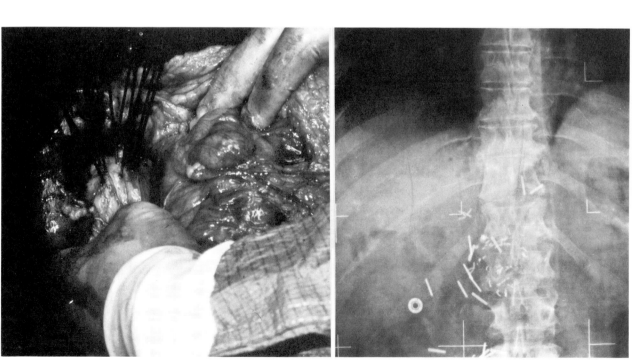

FIGURE 4-5

Classic Systems of Planning and Evaluation

In either the Manchester or the Quimby system, the planning of an interstitial implant consists of determining the area or volume of a target region and then referring to a table or graph for the required total source strength (milligram hour) per unit peripheral dose (1000 cGy) or, alternatively, the source activity for a given peripheral dose rate.

The objective of the interstitial *Manchester System* is to deliver a homogeneous dose, within plus or minus 10 percent of the prescribed dose, throughout the implanted region or in the 0.5-cm plane for planar implants, except for the localized high spots around each source. To achieve this "homogeneous" radiation, detailed source distribution rules specify a nonuniform source strength distribution between the target periphery and the target central region (**Table 4-1**).

The *Quimby System*, on the other hand, called for uniform distribution of source strength and accepted the resulting peaking of dose in the central implant region. For volume implants, the Quimby system prescribed dose was the same as the peripheral dose, which together with the central peaking, resulted in substantially higher integral dose, than in the Manchester system, for a given dose. Very large implants of uniformly spaced sources might be expected to have broad central regions of homogeneous dose, within 5 percent to Manchester system tables.

The *Paris System* was designed for implants of parallel line sources, such as Ir-192 wires. The average of doses calculated at points midway between source lines in the central transverse plane is defined as the *basal dose*. The isodose contour associated with 85 percent of the basal dose is specified as the treatment region periphery (the 0.6 Gy/h contour in **Fig. 4-6**). The treatment region dimensions depend on the spacing, number, and length of the radioactive sources (wires) in the implant, but not on the source strength. In **Fig. 4-7**, four 6-cm lines at 1-cm spacing serve to treat a region about 4.3-cm long, 3.7-cm wide, and 0.6-cm thick. Variations in dose rate are accomplished only by proportionate variations in source strength.

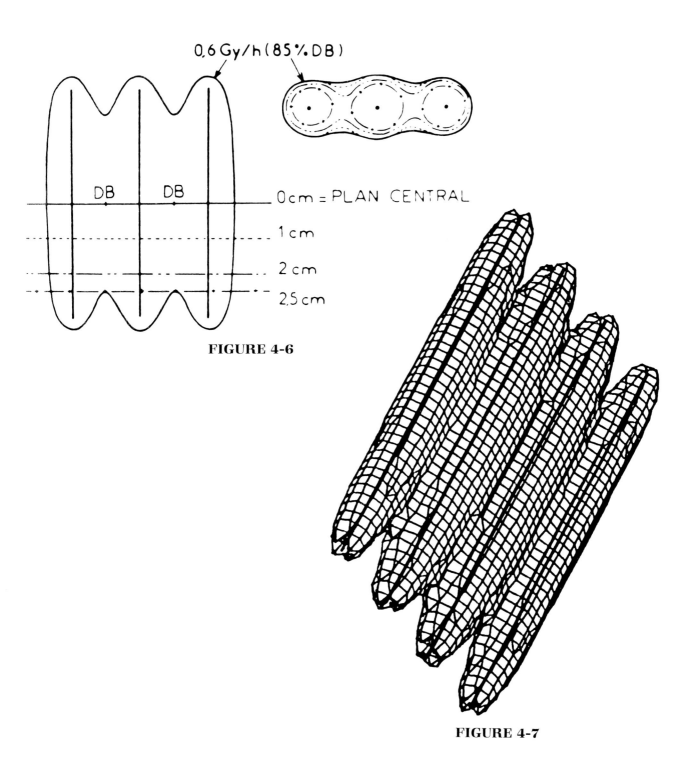

0.6 Gy/h (85% DB)

DB   DB

0 cm = PLAN CENTRAL

1 cm

2 cm

2.5 cm

FIGURE 4-6

FIGURE 4-7

TABLE 4-1. Manchester System Distribution Rules

	Region	Peripheral Fraction
Planar	< 25 cm²	⅔
	25–100 cm²	½
	> 100 cm²	⅓
Volume		¾

75

THE NEW YORK SYSTEM—TREATMENT PLANNING

With the increasing use of modern 3-D imaging techniques to aid brachytherapy procedures, it is clear that we are in a transitional period with respect to interstitial treatment planning. Ideally, our goal should be to optimize the strength and location arrangement of sources to produce the closest possible approach to a prescribed dose at all points on the periphery of the target region. Initial steps have already been taken toward the realization of such a goal by *least squares* optimization in certain treatment situations. Existing techniques make extensive use of nomographs developed in New York at Memorial Sloan-Kettering Cancer Center.

Temporary Implants

The Planar Implant Nomograph (**Fig. 4-8**). Although developed for implants of Ir-192 ribbons, this is applicable as well to other radionuclides, i.e., since source strength is taken to be in milligram-radium-equivalents (pending implementation of air–kerma strength units), and since simple inverse square attenuation is assumed, it is in no way specific to a particular radionuclide.

The reference dose is specified in the plane 0.5 cm distant from the source plane (**Fig. 4-9**) at points midway between outermost ribbons and 1.5 cm from the end seed centers inside the implanted region. For the 8 × 4 cm target area given in the example, the nomograph indicates that 5 lines of 9 seeds each will provide the closest approach to a 10 Gy/day dose rate at the reference points. Reference points defined in this manner, together with the uniform (Quimby-type) source spacing, require about the same total activity per unit dose as the Manchester system table for small areas, and about 14 percent more at an area of 100 cm².

The nomograph is intended to assist in the planning of surgical field (tumor bed) implants and of tumors about 1-cm thick.

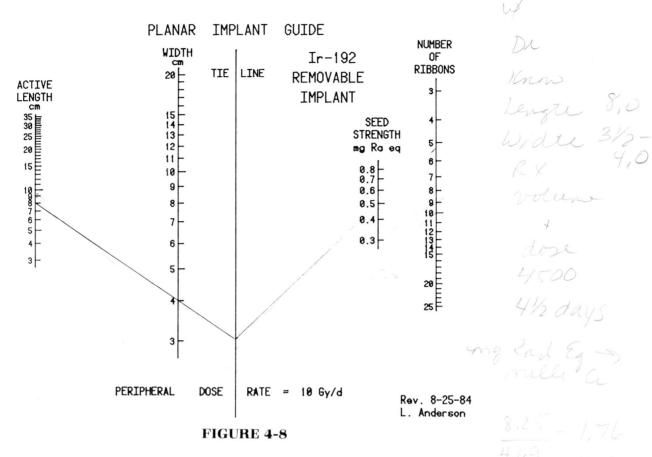

PLANAR IMPLANT GUIDE

FIGURE 4-8

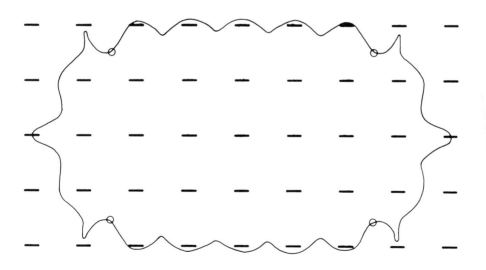

Isodose-Rate Contour
at Reference Point Dose Rate (9.3 Gy/d)

(0.5 cm PLANE)

8 cm × 4 cm   Specified optimum = 10 Gy/d

FIGURE 4-9

Extension of the nomographic method to implant planning in three dimensions presents operational complexity because of the many scales required.

The Two-Plane Nomograph (**Fig. 4-10**).   This was initially developed for breast implants. Other sites suitable for two-plane implants are the tongue, floor of the mouth, buccal mucosa, chest wall, and extremities. The nomograph assumes that the separation between the two planes is 1.5 cm and that the Ir-192 ribbons in the superficial plane are staggered and one fewer in number relative to those of the base-plane.

The reference point (**Fig. 4-11**) is defined for planar implants, but in the midplane 0.75 cm from each source plane.

In clinical use, the two-plane nomograph is similar to the planar nomograph in that it affords planning to achieve a given dose at a peripheral point defined in relation to the source lines themselves with no assumption regarding target region *thickness.* For idealized implants as large as the example in Figs. 4-10 and 4-11, the thickness of the 10 Gy/day contour (selected because of smoothness of contour and continuity of coverage) at the center of the implant is 3.5 cm, i.e., beyond the usual 1.5- to 2.5-cm range of target thickness for which two planes are recommended. In practice, for closely uniform spacing of source lines, the 1000 cGy/day isodose contour near the implant center is increasingly distant from the sources as the implanted area becomes larger, and treatment dose rate selections are commonly made at 1500 to 1600 cGy/day contours. If it is desired to treat at a certain dose rate to a specified thickness, spacings other than 1.5 cm should be considered.

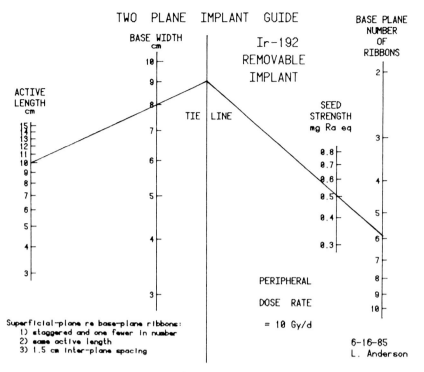

TWO PLANE IMPLANT GUIDE

BASE WIDTH
cm

Ir-192
REMOVABLE
IMPLANT

BASE PLANE
NUMBER
OF
RIBBONS

ACTIVE
LENGTH
cm

TIE LINE

SEED
STRENGTH
mg Ra eq

PERIPHERAL

DOSE RATE

= 10 Gy/d

Superficial-plane re base-plane ribbons:
1) staggered and one fewer in number
2) same active length
3) 1.5 cm inter-plane spacing

6-16-85
L. Anderson

FIGURE 4-10

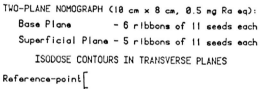

TWO-PLANE NOMOGRAPH (10 cm x 8 cm, 0.5 mg Ra eq):
   Base Plane   - 6 ribbons of 11 seeds each
   Superficial Plane - 5 ribbons of 11 seeds each

ISODOSE CONTOURS IN TRANSVERSE PLANES

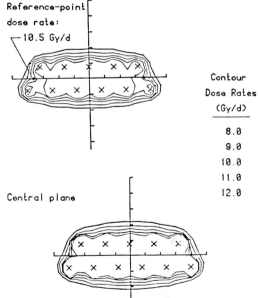

Reference-point
dose rate:

—10.5 Gy/d

Contour
Dose Rates
(Gy/d)

8.0
9.0
10.0
11.0
12.0

Central plane

FIGURE 4-11

In planning for *temporary volume implants,* i.e. when three dimensions of a target region have been specified or, better, when a 3-D target contour has been defined from CT or magnetic resonance imaging (MRI) scans, the current approach at Memorial is to "hand tailor" the dose distribution by repeated adjustments of the source distribution. This process is simplified and expedited with computer-assisted "building" of input data files containing trial arrays of sources. An example is our file-building program for multiplane implants, outlined in **Table 4-2**. This program quickly simulates individually dimensioned parallel planes of seeds in ribbons, with the entire structure automatically centered in all three coordinate axes.

A stepping-source remote afterloader makes feasible the *least-square optimization* to achieve good approximations to specified dose distributions. Results of this type of optimization are shown in **Table 4-3** for a planar array of six source lines with eight source positions per line. Because uniform dose is specified in the (0.5 cm distant) treatment plane, a symmetrical distribution is anticipated and target points midway between source positions need be specified only in one quadrant.

TABLE 4-2. Computer Simulation of Source Configuration for Rapid Planning of Two-Plane Temporary Implant

Enter:	Seed spacing *(cm)* along lines
	Number of planes
	Plane spacing
Enter plane 1	Number of seeds per line
	Number of lines
	Line spacing *(cm)*
Enter plane 2	Number of seeds per line
	Number of lines
	Line spacing *(cm)*

TABLE 4-3. GAMMA MED II: Optimized Planar Application 7 Gy Target at Points (*) in 0.5-cm Plane with Balanced Source-Plane Uniformity (Source: 10 Ci Ir-192)

Dwell-Time (s)   1.2 cm

9.9	*	8.3	*	8.1	*	8.1	8.3	9.9
6.8	*	5.3	*	5.0	*	5.0	5.3	6.8
6.8	*	5.1	*	4.9	*	4.9	5.1	6.8
6.7	*	5.1	*	4.9	*	4.9	5.1	6.7
6.7		5.1		4.9		4.9	5.1	6.7
6.8		5.1		4.9		4.9	5.1	6.8
6.8		5.3		5.0		5.0	5.3	6.8
9.9		8.3		8.1		8.1	8.3	9.9

1 cm

Dose (Gy) at Points (*)

Source Plane				*Treatment Plane*		
9.49	9.36	9.35		6.66	6.77	6.80
9.18	9.04	9.00		6.96	7.07	7.09
9.11	8.94	8.93		6.97	7.08	7.11
9.10	8.96	8.95		6.99	7.10	7.14
Coeff Vaf = 0.021				Coeff Var = 0.021		

Permanent Implants

The Memorial Nomograph for Iodine-125 Volume Implant. This began as a guide for seed spacing in implementing the original average dimension method of total source-strength specification. In the current nomograph (**Fig. 4-12**), the original rule, giving total (apparent) activity in millicuries as five times the average dimension in centimeters, is still used for average dimensions of 3.0 cm or less. For average dimensions of more than 3.0 cm, the total activity recommended is proportional to the 2.2 power of average dimension. Average dimension is determined by averaging three mutually perpendicular measured dimensions of the region to be treated. When elongation (largest–smallest dimension) is small (ratio < 1.5), the peripheral dose is expected to be approximately constant at 16,000 cGy for an average dimension equal to or more than 3.0 cm and inversely proportional to an average dimension for smaller implants. For larger elongations the nomograph overestimates the idealized activity requirement by a few percent.

The use of the I-125 permanent implant nomograph is illustrated in Fig. 4-12. To determine the number of I-125 sources required for the implant, draw a straight line from the *average dimension* to the *seed strength*. This line intersects the *number of seeds* scale and indicates the number of required seeds. To determine the spacing between needles for the I-125 implant, draw a straight line from number of seeds through the average dimension to *tie line*. From the point of intersection with the tie line a final line is drawn through the *spacing along needle* of the sources to *spacing between needles*. The number of sources per needle is determined from the selected spacing along needles and the average depth of the implant. The number of needles required for the implant is determined by dividing the total number of I-125 seeds required for the implant by the number of sources per needle.

For permanent as well as temporary implants the ultimate optimization goal is to bring treatment dose and target dose contours into coincidence. A specialized file-building algorithm facilitates planning from CT images. Deep source points within the target volume not necessarily in the same CT scan are identified for each needle. Seeds are distributed among target candidate locations at 0.5-cm intervals along each needle in sufficient number to provide the total strength recommended by the nomograph. The computer then supplies the 3-D coordinates of all seeds and permits checking the adequacy of dose distribution for a given trial. **Figure 4-13** illustrates percutaneous I-125 seed implants of lung tumors, a needle configuration planned to accomodate the presence of a rib preventing access to one-half of the target region.

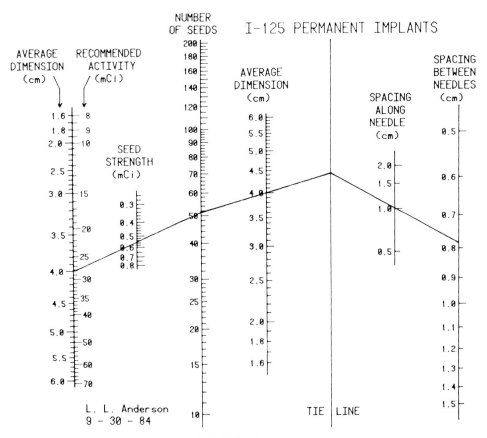

FIGURE 4-12

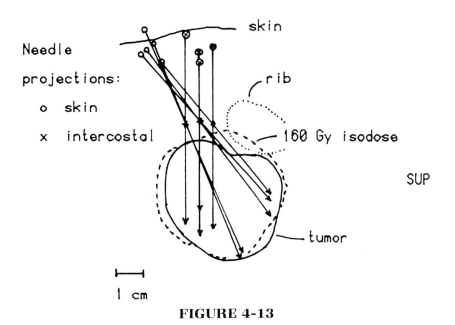

FIGURE 4-13

Dose Prescription

As will be detailed for specific sites in subsequent chapters, the dose prescription must take into account prior treatment, dose rate, treatment volume, and the tolerance of adjacent normal tissue, as well as tumor radiosensitivity. Early users of the Manchester System typically prescribed a dose that was equivalent to about 6400 cGy in a period of 6 to 8 days. A somewhat lower dosage was used for a substantially higher dose rate or for an unusually large volume.

For previously untreated tumors, it is generally accepted today that temporary-implant doses in the range of 6000 to 7000 cGy can be safely delivered in 6 to 7 days to treatment volumes of about 40 cc or smaller. Lower target doses are given in the case of either "boost" implant therapy in conjunction with external beam therapy or "tumor bed" treatment of microscopic disease in conjunction with surgery. For dose-rate variations in the range of 30 to 60 cGy/hour, many radiation oncologists do not make adjustments in the total dose prescribed. **Figure 4-14** shows the 3-D minimum target dose distribution for a planar implant (5 × 3 cm) using the New York System of dosimetry. The recommended full-treatment dose for permanent implants with I-125 (60-day half-life) is considered to lie between 14,000 and 18,000 cGy. **Figure 4-15** shows the 3-D minimum peripheral dose distribution for such an I-125 volume implant. Reductions in total dose may be indicated for larger volumes or if adjacent normal tissues have low radiation tolerance.

TREATMENT EVALUATION

Physical evaluation of a brachytherapy procedure ideally implies a comparison between doses planned at specified target points and doses actually achieved at the same points. Intrinsic in the evaluation process is the accurate calculation of each source's contribution to the dose at a point, making use of appropriate single-source reference data (see Chap. 1). Essential to such calculations is knowledge of the distance, and perhaps orientation, of each source with respect to the point of interest; localization methods will be discussed at the end of this chapter.

The distinction between planning and evaluation may become insignificant in certain types of procedures, e.g., when afterloading catheters are placed in a fixed, known relationship to target contours and final planning consists of optimizing the source "loading" within them.

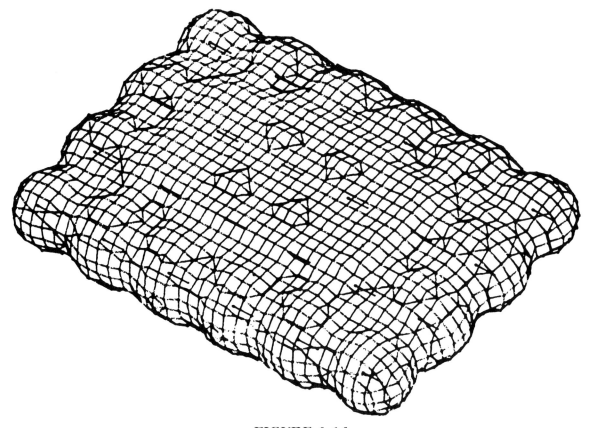

FIGURE 4-14

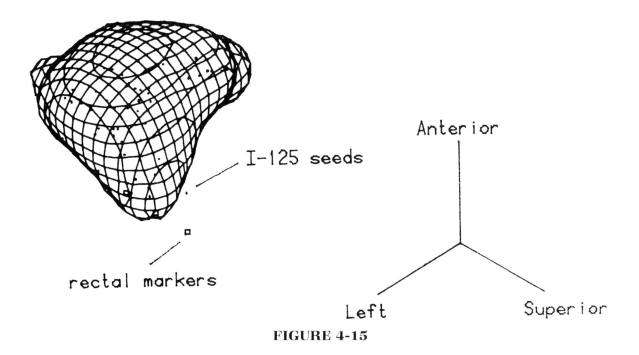

I-125 seeds

rectal markers

Anterior

Left

Superior

FIGURE 4-15

Evaluation of Temporary Implants

When temporary implants are performed to treat the "tumor bed" follow-ing tumor excision, the aim is to eradicate any microscopic disease on or between tissue surfaces that have been closed over the afterloading cathe-ters. Ideally, although the target may be represented as a zero-thickness plane or curved surface, in practice the tissue surfaces penetrate the "implant (source) plane" somewhat randomly, and the planar implant nomograph in catheter spacing, by planning for a 1.0-cm treatment-region thickness at reference points near the "corners" of the implant. The man-ner in which evaluation to determine treatment time is performed is illus-trated in **Fig. 4-16**:

- the heavy-lined inner continuous isodose contour (centigray/day) for each of several standard computer planes is selected as the highest dose-rate contour for which there are no gaps within the target region.
- the median peripheral dose-rate (MPDR) contour is determined from the preceding (e.g., 900 cGy/day). *10 Gy/day*
- the recommended median peripheral dose (MPD) for the particular implant is prescribed (e.g., 4500 cGy).
- the MPD in centigray is divided by the MPDR in centigray/day to deter-mine the treatment time in days, (e.g., 5 days, in our example, to deliver the prescribed dose of 4500 cGy).

10 cgy/day
4500 in
4.5 days

Also part of the evaluation for this patient was the determination of sat-isfactorily normal tissue dose (e.g., skin, spinal cord, rectum, etc.).

Evaluation of temporary *volume implants* entails either comparing dose rates achieved with dose rate intended at specified target points or, alter-natively, identifying a dose rate for which the isodose contour adequately encloses the target. The latter approach was adopted in evaluating the dose distribution for the template-guided Ir-192 implant shown in Fig. 4-17 (left), where the 1000 cGy/day contour was selected as adequately encompassing the CT-defined target. In either approach, the treatment dose rate is decided and is then used to determine the treatment time. For the perirectal tumor treatment of **Fig. 4-17** (right) a dose of 3000 cGy was delivered in 3 days.

Since treatment time is determined as a result of these analyses, one may contend that they constitute planning as much as evaluation. Again, the dis-tinction is important mainly for discussion purposes, and the essential con-sideration regarding evaluation is that we know how the dose was actually delivered.

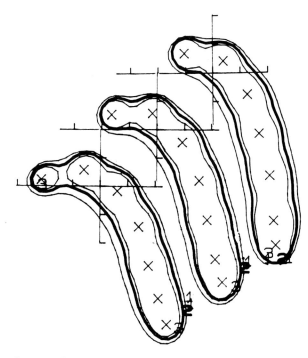

Treatment Dose-Rate Selection
FIGURE 4-16

- - - - target contour

--------- rectal obturator

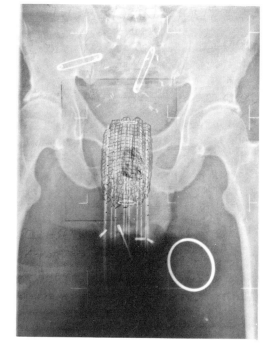

FIGURE 4-17

87

Evaluation of Permanent Implants

Although isodose contours may no longer be manipulated once a permanent implant has been performed, a thorough evaluation of the dose distribution obtained is nevertheless important both to further management of the patient and to ongoing quality assurance in comparable procedures. If accurate registration of the dose distribution is available with respect to 3-D anatomical images, it may be possible to determine the target region's minimum peripheral dose, which is generally accepted as the dose of greatest clinical significance. In many instances, however, 3-D images of the region are either lacking or fail to show clearly the target outline, and one must rely on the brachytherapist's having placed the sources in the correct region and having determined correctly the target dimensions. In such situations, the *matched peripheral dose* (MPD) can serve as a useful approximation to the *minimum peripheral dose* (MPD).

The matched peripheral dose is defined as the dose for which the contour volume is equal to the volume of an ellipsoid having the same dimensions as the measured, mutually perpendicular dimensions of the target region. It is determined, as illustrated in **Fig. 4-18**, by interpolating between computer calculated isodose contour volumes for various dose levels. Except in the unlikely event that both the target volume and the same-volume isodose contour are ellipsoidal, the target will project beyond the dose contour in some regions and recede within it in others. The matched peripheral dose will, therefore, generally be higher by a few percent than the true minimum peripheral dose.

Matched Peripheral Dose (MPD) from Dose Volume Data

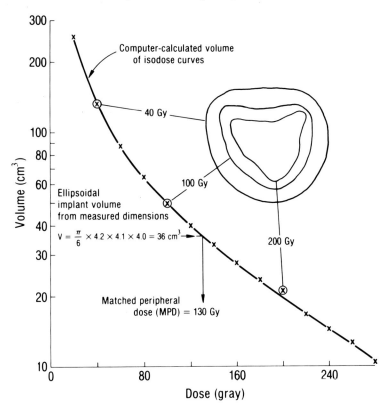

FIGURE 4-18

Volume–Dose Histograms

An important aspect of treatment evaluation in brachytherapy is the distribution of volume as a function of dose rate, particularly as it pertains to the question of dose uniformity and the relative position of the "treatment" dose rate. A simple plot of volume per unit dose rate versus dose rate, because of the inverse square law, produces a curve that is very high at low dose rates and low at high dose rates, and any interesting structure in between is largely obscured by the rapid fall-off. A more illuminating plot is one that supresses the inverse square effect. (Anderson, 1986)

In **Fig. 4-19**, the volume per unit $-\frac{3}{2}$ power of dose rate is plotted against the $-\frac{3}{2}$ power of the dose rate, and the plot for a point source (curve 1 in the figure), is a horizontal straight line. Splitting the total strength between two sources (curve 2) or among three sources (curve 3) 2 cm apart results in a volume "trapping" in regions midway between or among the sources; the dose rates in these regions correspond to the peaks in the histogram curves. These zones of near-constant dose rate are evident in the isodose patterns shown on the left.

In **Fig. 4-20** the total strength is split among multiple sources, resulting in sharply peaked histograms. Near perfect dose rate uniformity corresponds to a very high, narrow peak, while a very poor dose rate uniformity would be the horizontal line for the single source case (in Fig. 4-19). It has earlier been pointed out that only minor differences in uniformity exist between wire source implants and seed implants. (Anderson, 1985) For the wire or seed source arrangement of Fig. 4-20 to calculate "uniformity; 1) determine the treatment dose rate as per instructions on the left of Fig. 4-16 (i.e., 62 cGy/hour), mark the corresponding value on the histogram baseline and project it to the curve (line L); 2) determine the half-maximum dose rate value on the upper side of the peak and project it on the baseline (line H); 3) calculate the volume under the curve that falls between the treatment dose rate and the half-maximum dose rate (between lines L and H) by superimposing a graph paper and counting the number of squares; 4) calculate, in a similar way, the total treatment volume under the curve between line L and the end of the scale; 5) calculate the proportion of step 3 over step 4 (51 percent); 6) obtain the ratio of baseline distance between L and H and total baseline distance between L and end of scale (24 percent); 7) finally, divide the treatment volume proportion obtained in step 5 by the baseline distance proportion obtained in step 6 (51 percent/24 percent) to obtain the *uniformity value* (= 2.1).

The uniformity values obtained in clinical practice are in the range of 1.2 to 2.3. The higher the value the better the dose-rate uniformity.

The utility of volume–dose histograms to evaluate these and other implant parameters is currently under intensive investigation.

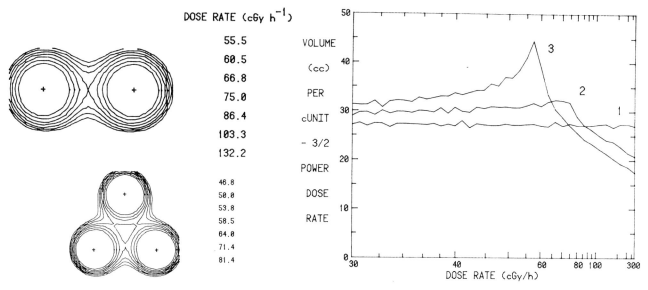

DOSE RATE (cGy h^{-1})

55.5
60.5
66.8
75.0
86.4
103.3
132.2

46.8
50.0
53.8
58.5
64.0
71.4
81.4

FIGURE 4-19

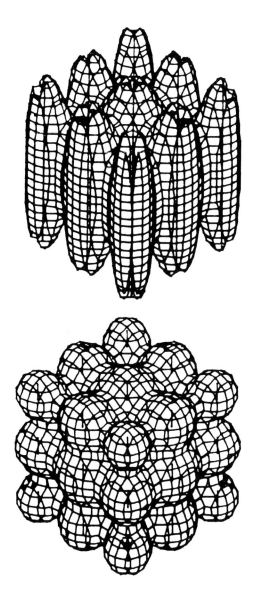

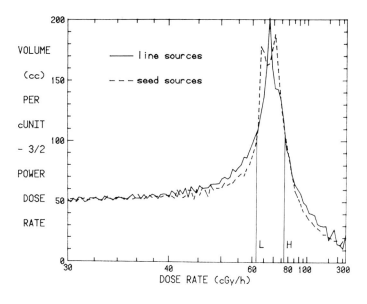

FIGURE 4-20

Source Localization

To specify the minimum dose rate to the target region requires careful localization of sources and computer calculation of the three-dimensional radiation dose distribution.

Orthogonal radiographs generally afford the most accurate and straightforward means of determining the distribution of implanted sources relative to one another, as long as the image of each source is identifiable in each film. The center of the implant is on a line that is perpendicular to the film, in each case, and passes through the x-ray tube target. Radiographic magnification is given by the ratio of target-film distance to target-implant distance. To determine the latter, it is helpful to place a strip of lead numbers on the surface of the patient, for each film, within but near the edge of the x-ray field. Variable magnification within extensive implants can be accommodated with an algorithm that makes use of localization data from a metal ring, seen, in the same position on the patient, in both films.

Stereo-shift films is a convenient alternative when image identification between orthogonal films is not possible (**Fig. 4-21**). The patient is shifted, usually longitudinally, a measured distance for a second anterioposterior film, without moving the x-ray tube. Coordinates in the anterioposterior direction are calculable because images of points farther from the film plane are shifted more between the two films than images of closer points.

Lateral-shift with angulation is used as an alternative to the orthogonal method for implants or applications in regions where bone structure may obscure images in a straight lateral or even a straight anterioposterior view (**Fig. 4-22**). The method combines the accuracy of the orthogonal method with the precision in identification of the stereo-shift method. The technique requires two oblique films taken from the right and left side of the radiological table at arbitrary angles—usually more than 15 degrees with respect to the normal table.

Computer-assisted image identification is readily possible using *three-film localization*, either based on isocentric geometry or requiring the use of a jig. Brachytherapy dosimetry is able to provide isodose contour overlays on CT scans, based on dose distributions computed from standard localization films. Localization of sources relative to anatomical features is all-important for improved registration accuracy between localization radiographs and CT (or MRI) scans are under active development. Reconstruction from scout-view source images would afford a direct method of achieving accurate registration.

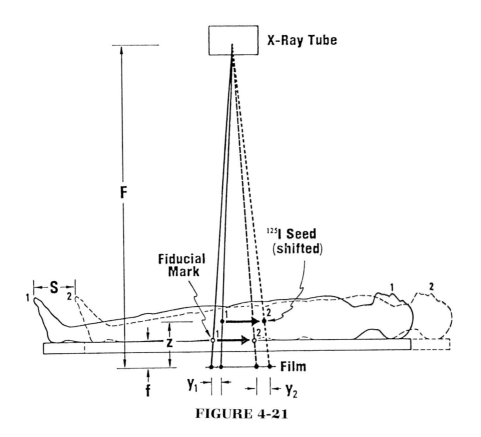

FIGURE 4-21

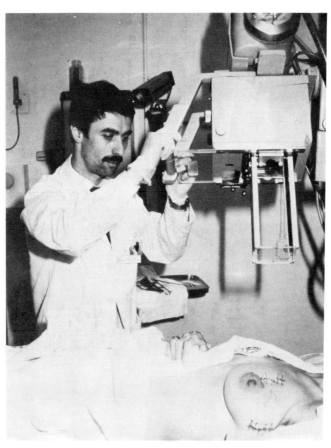

FIGURE 4-22

REFERENCES

1. Meredith, W. J., ed. *Radiation dosage, the Manchester System*, Second Edition. Edinburgh: E. & S. Livingstone, 1967. p. 134.

2. Glasser, O, Quimby, E. H., Taylor, L. S., Weatherwax, J. L., and Morgan, R. H. *Physical Foundations of Radiology*. Third edition. New York: Harper and Row, 1961. p. 503.

3. Shalek, R. J., Stovall, M. A., and Sampiere, V. A. The radiation distribution and dose specification in volume implants of radioactive seeds. *Am J Roentgenol* 77:863–868, 1957.

4. Dutreix, A., Marinello, G., and Wambersie, A. Dosimetrie en curietherapie. Paris: Masson, 1982. p. 277.

5. Anderson, L. L., Hilaris, B. S., and Wagner, L. K. A nomograph for planar implant planning. *Endocuriether Hyperthermia Oncol* 1:9–15, 1985.

6. Anderson, L. L., and Osian, A. D. Brachytherapy optimization and evaluation. *Endocuriether Hyperthermia Oncol* 2S:25–32, 1986.

7. Anderson, L. L. Treatment optimization with the Gamma Med II. In: Mick, F. W. (ed): *Proceedings of the First Symposium on Gamma-Med Remote Afterloading; 1985 May 11, Washington DC.* New York: Mick Radio-Nuclear Instruments, Inc. 1985, pp. 18–27.

8. Anderson, L. L. Spacing nomograph for interstitial implants of 125 I seeds. *Med Phys* 3:48–51, 1976.

9. Henschke, U. K., and Cevc, P. Dimension averaging, a simple method for dosimetry of interstitial implants. *Radiobiol Radiother* 9:287–298, 1968.

10. Anderson, L. L., and Osian, A. Radionuclides, instrumentation and computerized dosimetry. In: Hilaris, B. S., and Nori, D. (eds): *Brachytherapy Oncology Update—1984.* New York: Memorial Sloan-Kettering Cancer Center, 1984, pp. 13–18.

11. Anderson, L. L. Physical optimization of afterloading techniques. *Strahlentherapie* 161:264–269, 1985.

12. Heelan, R. T., Hilaris, B. S., Anderson, L. L., Nori, D., Martini, N., Wabon, R. C. Caravelli, J. F., and Linares, L. A. Percutaneous I-125 source implantation of lung tumors with computed tomographic treatment planning: early experience. *Radiology* 164:735–740, 1987.

13. Anderson, L. L. A "natural" volume-dose histogram for brachytherapy. *Med Phys* 13:898–903, 1986.

14. Paul, J. M., Koch, R. F., Philip, P. C., and Khan, F. R. Uniformity of dose distribution in interstitial implants. *Endocuriether Hyperthermia Oncol* 2:107–118, 1986.

15. Wu, A., and Sternick, E. S. A dose homogeneity index for evaluating Ir-192 interstitial breast implants. *Med Phys* 14: (in press), 1987.

16. Anderson, L. L. Dose homogeneity in seed line source implants. *J Int Fed Medical and Biological Engineering* 23 (Suppl Part 2, Proc XVI Int Conf on Medical and Biological Engineering and VII Int Conf on Medical Physics): 1180–1181, 1985.

17. Anderson, L. L. Dosimetry for interstitial radiation therapy. In: Hilaris, B. S. (ed.): *Handbook of interstitial brachytherapy.* Acton, Mass.: Publishing Sciences Group, 1975, pp. 87–115.

18. Mohan, R., and Anderson, L. L. *Brachy II Interstitial and Intracavitary Dose Computation Program User's Guide.* New York: Memorial Sloan-Kettering Cancer Center, 1982.

19. Thomadsen, B. R., and Shahabi, S. Video tape recording assistance in radiotherapy seed identification (Abstr.). *Med Phys* 14:476 May/June 1987.

20. Anderson, L. L., Kuan, H. M., and Ding, I. Y. Clinical dosimetry with 125 I. In: George, F. W. (ed.): *Modern Interstitial and Intracavitary Radiation Cancer Management*. New York: Masson Publishing USA, 1981, pp. 9–15.

21. Sharma, S. C., Williamson, J. F., and Cytacki, E. Dosimetric analysis of stereo and orthogonal reconstruction of interstitial implants. *Int J Radiat Oncol Biol Phys* 8:1803–1805, 1982.

22. Hilaris, B. S., Nori, D., and Anderson, L. L. Brachytherapy treatment planning. In: Vaeth, J. M., and Meyer, J. (eds.): *Treatment Planning in the Radiation Therapy of Cancer, Frontiers of Radiation Therapy and Oncology*, Vol. 21. Basel: Karger, 1987, pp. 94–106.

23. Amols, H. I., and Rosen, I. I. A three-film technique for reconstruction of radioactive seed implants. *Med Phys* 8:210–214, 1981.

24. Rosenthal, M. S., and Nath, R. An automatic seed identification technique for interstitial implants using three isocentric radiographs. *Med Phys* 10:475–479, 1983.

25. Biggs, P. J., and Kelley, D. M. Geometric reconstruction of seed implants using a three-film technique. *Med Phys* 10:701–704, 1983.

26. Jackson, D. D. An automatic method for localizing radioactive seeds in implant dosimetry. *Med Phys* 10:370–372, 1983.

27. Altschuler, M. D., Findlay, P. A., and Epperson, R. D. Rapid, accurate, three-dimensional location of multiple seeds in implant radiotherapy treatment planning. *Phys Med Biol* 28:1305–1318, 1983.

28. Siddon, R. L., and Chin, L. M. Two-film brachytherapy reconstruction algorithm. *Med Phys* 12:77–83, 1985.

29. Rosen, I. I., Khan, K. M., Lane, R. G., and Kelsey, C. A. The effect of geometric errors in the reconstruction of iridium-192 seed implants. *Med Phys* 9:220–223, 1982.

CHAPTER 5

Intracavitary Brachytherapy Planning and Evaluation

The introduction of an afterloading applicator by Henschke in 1960 to treat cervix cancer made it possible to plan radiation dose distributions for such treatments in relation to anatomical features established radiographically prior to source loading. Thus, to the extent that an intracavitary applicator may be assumed to maintain its initial geometry throughout treatment, evaluation of the dose distribution will have been accomplished once the planning is complete. In general, this merger of planning and evaluation has been more evident for intracavitary radiotherapy, where planning has consisted of rearranging sources within predetermined pathways than for interstitial therapy, where selection of pathways has been the major part of the planning, and evaluation has focused on pathways realized. Since 1976, source-configuration adjustments for cervix applicators at Memorial Hospital have been performed using least-squares optimization techniques, and since 1984 these methods have involved dose calculations based on 3-D lookup tables to take asymmetrical ovoid shields (see **Fig. 5-1**) into account.

Intracavitary treatments differ further from interstitial treatments in that sources are generally larger and less likely to be in direct contact with tissue. Dose calculations must take account of interposed materials as well as of the effects of the source encapsulation itself. In contrast to the seeds used in interstitial therapy, where geometrical attenuation is well approximated by the inverse square law, intracavitary sources usually involve a spatial distribution of radioactivity that, for calculating geometrical attenuation, may be approximated by a straight line (see **Fig. 5-2**). Lookup tables are more manageable (less variable data, permitting linear interpolation in a shorter table) if the quantity tabulated is proportional not just to the dose rate, but to the dose rate divided by geometrical attentuation; for line sources, the geometrical attenuation is a function of the active length and orientation as well as distance, as depicted in the figure.

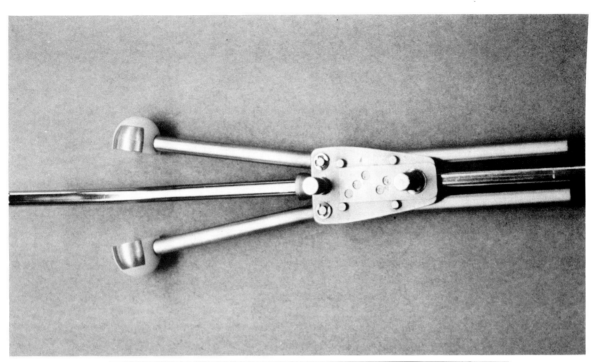

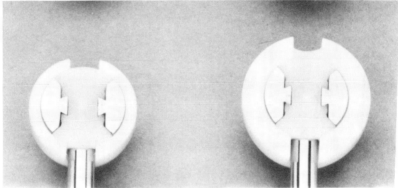

FIGURE 5-1

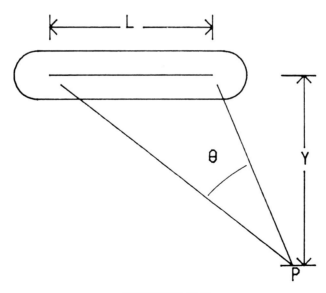

FIGURE 5-2

CLASSICAL METHODOLOGY FOR CERVIX CANCER

The most extensive application of intracavitary brachytherapy has been in the treatment of uterine cervix cancer, for which the use of radium was reported as early as 1903. Well-defined systems for such treatments had evolved by 1920 at radium centers in Stockholm and Paris. In the Stockholm system, source strengths were high and treatment times were short relative to the Paris system; the Manchester technique, described in 1938, involved intermediate values of source strength and treatment time (see **Fig. 5-3**).

The Manchester approach differed significantly from the earlier system in that treatments were no longer specified simply in milligram-hours, but in terms of quantity now called exposure, in *roentgen units*, at points of interest representing anatomical features. In particular, the treatment dose was specified at "Point A," 2 cm lateral to the center of the uterine canal and 2 cm (along a line parallel to the uterine axis) from the lateral-fornix vaginal mucosa. This point was assumed close, on the average, to the location where the ureter crosses under the uterine artery; radiation necrosis in this region was taken as dose-limiting. A second point, "Point B," was defined to be 5 cm lateral to the patient's midline, at the same level as point A. Point B was assumed to be in or near to the obturator lymph node, the first node in a likely direction of disease extension, where the concern was that the dose be adequate.

The Manchester applicator consisted of a thin rubber intrauterine tube, in lengths to accommodate one, two, or three radium tubes (2.2-cm long) according to the length of the uterus, and a pair of rubber vaginal *ovoids* (each containing a single radium tube), with diameters of 2.0, 2.5, or 3.0 cm. The roughly ellipsoidal shape of the ovoids was selected to match the shape of the radium dose contours and enhance surface uniformity. Ovoids were separated, if possible, by a 1-cm spacer or, for narrow vaginas, merely held in juxtaposition by a washer. The assembled components were packed into position with one ovoid in each fornix and the ovoid sources perpendicular both to the line joining their centers and to the uterine sources.

A typical Point A dose in the Manchester system was 4000 R in each of two sessions, separated by a 4 to 7 day rest period, at a dose rate of about 57 R/hour. To limit the dose to the vaginal mucosa, the contribution of vaginal sources to the dose at Point A was restricted to less than about 40 percent of the total (see **Fig. 5-4**). The Point B dose rate depends mainly on the total source strength and is about one-third of the Point A dose for the loading indicated in the figure caption.

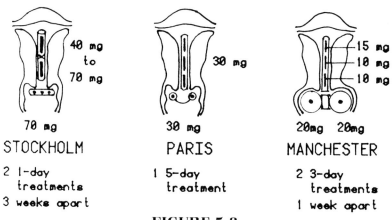

FIGURE 5-3

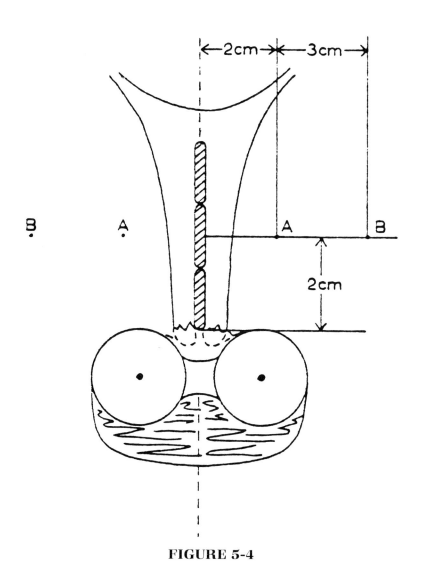

FIGURE 5-4

NEW YORK SYSTEM OF DOSIMETRY

The New York System, developed at Memorial Sloan-Kettering Cancer Center, has been patterned after the Manchester system, with a treatment-dose reference point definition closely analogous to that of the Manchester Point A. The New York system's specification of other treatment and tolerance points, together with corresponding dose objectives, are tabulated in Chap. 14 and illustrated diagrammatically in **Fig. 5-5**. Tolerance points are those for which the target dose is given as an upper limit. The desired dose rate at the reference point is 60 cGy/hour.

In the New York system, optimization of the dose distribution has been performed by repeated adjustments of source strengths at "dummy" source locations determined from orthogonal films taken prior to loading. For more than 10 years, this process has been computer-assisted, using an iterative algorithm developed by Rosenstein. Treatment points are readily visualized in the A/P radiographic projection (see Fig. 5-5). In addition to the reference points (REF), the optimization process includes uterine surface points (UTE), cervix points (CVX), and vaginal surface points (VG$_1$). Other points of interest shown, for which the dose is merely recorded, are vaginal points at a depth of 0.5 cm (VG$_2$) and obturator node points (OBT), which are close to Manchester Point B. Tissue tolerance points are best shown in the lateral projection (see Fig. 5-5). Tolerance points included in optimization are five rectal probe points (R$_{1-5}$), a bladder point (BL$_1$) in the center of the Foley catheter balloon, and a sigmoid colon point (SC) midway between the applicator tip and the sacral promontorium. Also, dose is recorded at a bladder point (BL$_2$) on the Foley balloon surface.

Optimization by computer begins with the assumption that all candidate source locations contain the same source strength (see **Table 5-1**) and by evaluating a *minimization parameter*, the sum of squares of differences between desired and obtained doses at included points. Systematic replacement of source strengths at each location with actual strengths available, reevaluating the minimization parameter after each change, and retaining the strength that gives a minimum, results in the strength distribution for iteration #1. Subsequent iterations lead quickly to a configuration that repeats and is taken as optimum. Doses achieved, normalized to doses desired, generally show a standard deviation of 8 to 12 percent.

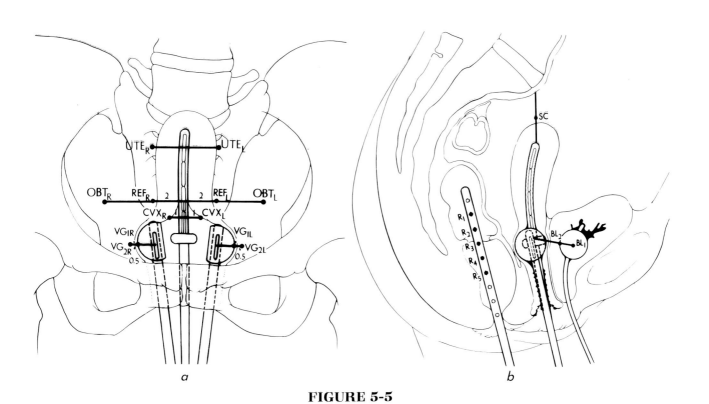

a

b

FIGURE 5-5

TABLE 5-1

Iteration	Minimization Parameter	Source strengths (mg Ra eq)					
		Tandem			Ovoids		
0	0.01740	10.0	10.0	10.0	10.0	10.0	10.0
1	0.00592	15.9	4.1	6.3	10.4	12.1	12.1
2	0.00524	15.9	6.3	4.1	10.4	12.1	12.1
3	0.00451	15.9	8.0	4.1	12.1	12.1	12.1
4	0.00451	15.9	8.0	4.1	12.1	12.1	12.1

THE HENSCHKE APPLICATOR

In order to realize satisfactory dose optimization among points of interest in cervix applications, i.e., in order to deliver a prescribed reference-point treatment dose with an acceptably low dose at tolerance points, it is essential that the applicator be properly inserted and that its design allow a favorable geometry. To obtain the lowest ratio between rectal dose and reference-point (point A) dose, for example, it is important that vaginal sources be inserted as far as possible and be spread as far as possible. The extent to which these objectives are met will depend on the shape of the vaginal colpostats.

Figure 5-6 illustrates the relative merits of a 2-cm-diameter cylindrical and a 2.5-cm-diameter hemispherical (ovoid) colpostat—the sizes most used clinically in Fletcher and Henschke type applicators, respectively. On the left side of the drawing, which shows a lateral view of insertion in the (nominally) superior direction, it is evident that the center of the colpostat, which is also the center of the source, is 0.5 cm more superior for the hemispherical than for the cylindrical shape. The criterion here is simply one of equal perimeters of tissue in contact with the colpostat in a plane parallel to the sagittal plane. The question of colpostat spreading is considered in the transverse view on the right side of Fig. 5-6. The spreads shown, 3.4 cm between centers for the cylinders and 4.4 cm for the ovoids, are those that result in 16.6-cm perimeters in the transverse plane for each case. Although these criteria are idealized, it is clear that the hemispherical colpostat shown has a distinct advantage over its cylindrical counterpart.

A comparison between the Henschke applicator and a Fletcher-type applicator is shown in **Fig. 5-7**. The data for the Fletcher-type applicator have been taken, without modification, from a similar published comparison for which unrealistic Henschke data were used (Delclos et al., 1978). The Henschke applicator data here are for 2.5-cm diameter ovoids (rather than 2.0 cm, as in the earlier comparison), which is the diameter used in nearly all clinical applications at Memorial Hospital. Moreover, the ovoid spread has been increased (from 3.2 cm in the earlier comparison) to 3.9 cm, which is the average of the value that results in a transverse perimeter equal to that of the Fletcher cylinders and the value that results in the same area enclosed by the transverse perimeter. Finally, tungsten shields not considered earlier have now been included and have been accounted for in the dose calculations. In this more realistic comparison, comparable doses for the two applicator types are found at midline points representing the bladder and rectum, and the dose at points 0.5 cm directly anterior or posterior to the colpostats is 22 percent lower for the Henschke applicator (Anderson et al., 1987).

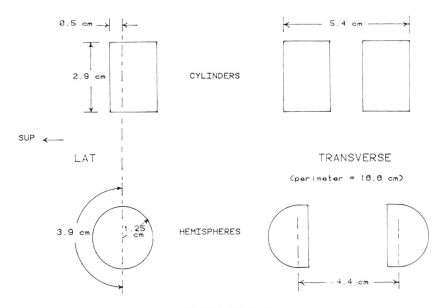

FIGURE 5-6

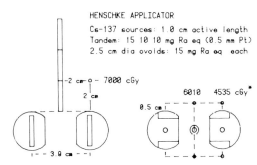

HENSCHKE APPLICATOR

Cs-137 sources: 1.0 cm active length
Tandem: 15 10 10 mg Ra eq (0.5 mm Pt)
2.5 cm dia ovoids: 15 mg Ra eq each

* Doses based on 3D measurements for shielded ovoids

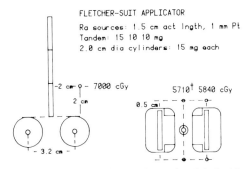

FLETCHER-SUIT APPLICATOR

Ra sources: 1.5 cm act lngth, 1 mm Pt
Tandem: 15 10 10 mg
2.0 cm dia cylinders: 15 mg each

† Includes 15% absorption from bladder and rectal shields

FIGURE 5-7

DOSE CALCULATION FOR SHIELDED OVOIDS

The tungsten inserts used in the 2-cm diameter Henschke ovoid (see Fig. 5-1) have a maximum shield thickness of about 6 mm. They are attached anteriorly and posteriorly on each ovoid by tongue-and-groove insertion from the medial side. The decision to incorporate shields was based on thermoluminescent dosimetry (TLD) measurements around an applicator in a water equivalent phantom at clinically typical locations of the points of interest used in the New York system (Masterson et al., 1982). Dose reductions of about 10 to 15 percent were observed at rectum and bladder points when the shields were used. The 2.5-cm diameter ovoid (and the 3.0-cm diameter, as well) is obtained by adding a snap-on nylon cap.

A secondary effect of adding the shields is to negate the cylindrical symmetry characteristic of a simple linear source's dose distribution, i.e., a 2-D lookup table is no longer feasible. In order to acquire the necessary 3-D data for a Cs-137 linear source in a shielded ovoid, extensive measurements in a water phantom were performed using a silicon diode detector (Mohan et al., 1985). Relative motions of the detector and source systems were obtained by stepping motors under computer control. The measurements were repeated for an unshielded ovoid to permit formulating a 3-D matrix of shielded/unshielded dose ratios. In the ratio data, possible error from energy or angular dependence of the diode is suppressed.

A final set of 3-D computer reference data was created by normalizing the unshielded relative diode data to a much smaller set of TLD measurements in a polystyrene phantom (Drozdoff et al., 1983). The LiF TLD chips used have significantly less energy and angular dependence than the diode, but involve a measurement technique not as readily automated. Both shielded and unshielded TLD measurements were made to permit comparison with the diode data and validation of the ratio approach. Excerpts from the TLD data are shown in **Fig. 5-8**, which gives dose ratios as a function of angle and distance from source center. The maximum attenuations observed are about 50 percent.

The 3-D dose reference data for shielded ovoid sources requires substantial changes in computational technique (Mohan et al., 1985). Most important is the necessity of three-point localization to specify shield orientation. Because the applicator yoke fixes orientation relative to the plane containing both sources, it is possible to define each ovoid source assembly by the two ends of the source plus one end of the other-ovoid source. Interpolation routines also require revision when three dimensions are involved; isodose surfaces for shielded and unshielded Cs-137 sources are compared at several dose levels in **Fig. 5-9**.

SHIELDED/UNSHIELDED RATIO OF TLD MEASUREMENTS IN
POLYSTYRENE PHANTOM AROUND CERVIX-APPLICATOR OVOID

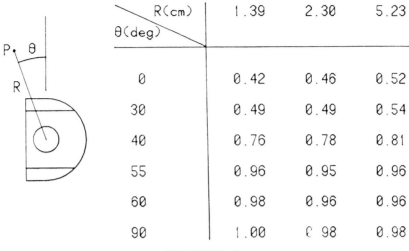

R(cm) θ(deg)	1.39	2.30	5.23
0	0.42	0.46	0.52
30	0.49	0.49	0.54
40	0.76	0.78	0.81
55	0.96	0.95	0.96
60	0.98	0.96	0.96
90	1.00	0.98	0.98

FIGURE 5-8

ISODOSE SURFACES FOR UNSHIELDED
AND SHIELDED SOURCE

Normalization Point: X= 2.1cm, Y= 0, Z= 0

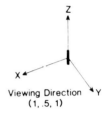

Viewing Direction
(1, .5, 1)

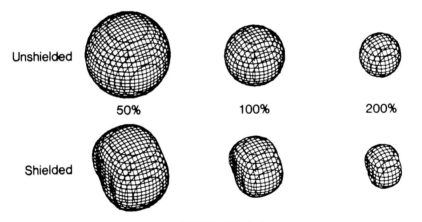

FIGURE 5-9

ICRU RECOMMENDATIONS FOR REPORTING

Regardless of the approach to planning intracavitary radiation therapy for cervix cancer, evaluation and comparison of clinical results will be more meaningful if a standard system is used in reporting the dose distribution. The International Commission on Radiation Units and Measurements (ICRU) has recently published recommendations for such standardized reporting (ICRU Report 38, 1985).

In addition to defining target volume and treatment volume (see Glossary), as shown in **Fig. 5-10**, the ICRU has defined, for reporting purposes, a *reference volume* as the volume enclosed by a reference isodose surface at an agreed-upon dose level, for which the recommended value is 60 Gy at low dose rates (0.4 to 2 Gy/hour) or an equivalent dose at higher dose rates. Isodose distributions used must include the total dose from all intracavitary applications and must include contours for 60 Gy in at least two planes (see **Fig. 5-11**) to facilitate determining mutually orthogonal reference-volume dimensions. The height (d_h) of the reference volume is measured along the uterine source line, and the width (d_w) and thickness (d_t) are measured along lines perpendicular to the length in the oblique frontal and sagittal planes, respectively. For combined intracavitary and external beam therapy, the reference-volume dose level is reduced by subtracting (from 60 Gy) the external beam dose, and the reference volume is, of course, increased.

Dose reporting is recommended at specific points, some of which represent organs and are close to the sources (which necessitates precise determination) and others of which are defined by bony structures and are farther from the sources. Practical definitions are given to allow locating points from orthogonal films. The rectal reference point, for example (see **Fig. 5-12**) is taken to be 0.5 cm posterior to the (opacified) posterior vaginal wall along an anterior/posterior (A/P) line, drawn on the lateral radiograph, through the lower end of the intrauterine source train. Similarly, the bladder reference point is set at the posterior surface of the opacified Foley balloon, along an A/P line drawn through its center.

Paraaortic, common iliac, and external iliac nodes are represented by reference points at the top, center, and bottom, respectively, of the sides of a *lymphatic trapezoid* with a 4-cm top at the center of L4 and a 12-cm base centered midway between the S1–S2 junction and the top of the symphysis. Also, a reference point representing each pelvic wall (and obturator node) is obtained at the intersection of horizontal and vertical lines drawn on the A/P radiograph, through the most superior and inner aspects, respectively, of the acetabulum and midway between the most superior acetabulum points on the lateral film.

Finally, in addition to reference-volume dimensions and specific reference-point doses, the ICRU recommends that reporting include the time–dose pattern, a complete description of technique (sources and applicator), and a statement of the total reference air–kerma (cumulated air–kerma strength).

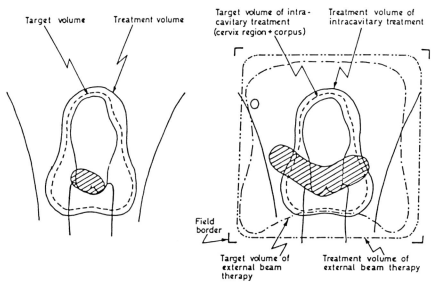

A. ONLY INTRACAVITARY TREATMENT

Target volume   Treatment volume

B. COMBINED INTRACAVITARY AND EXTERNAL BEAM THERAPY

Target volume of intra-cavitary treatment (cervix region + corpus)   Treatment volume of intracavitary treatment

Field border

Target volume of external beam therapy   Treatment volume of external beam therapy

FIGURE 5-10

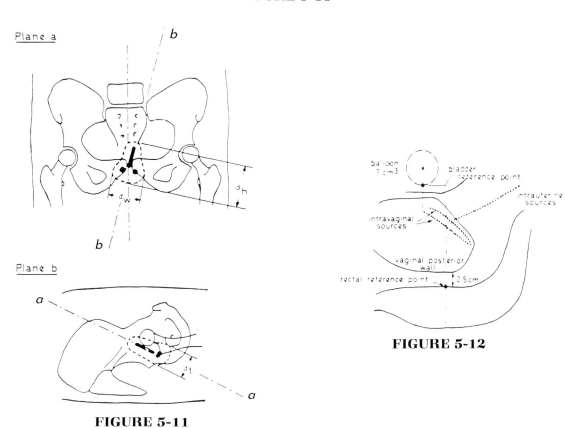

Plane a

b

b

Plane b

a

a

FIGURE 5-11

balloon 7 cm3   bladder reference point

intrauterine sources

intravaginal sources

vaginal posterior wall

rectal reference point   0.5 cm

FIGURE 5-12

OPTIMIZATION OF HIGH DOSE RATE REMOTE AFTERLOADER TREATMENTS

The stepping-source remote afterloader has introduced a new dimension in brachytherapy planning that makes possible an essentially complete selection of relative source-strength values, in contrast, for example, to the discrete source strengths available for optimizing conventional low dose rate afterloading, as discussed earlier. Typically, candidate source locations are distributed uniformly, at a specified increment, along one or more straight lines. The dwell-time of a cable-mounted source (e.g., 10 Ci Ir-192) at each of these applicator locations is, in effect, the source strength for planning purposes.

For a relatively simple application involving a single line of sources and an equal number of uniform-dose specification points along a line parallel to the source line (see **Fig. 5-13**) it may be possible to obtain the desired doses exactly. In the figure, exactly 5 Gy at all seven points of interest is mathematically possible for treatment distances ranging from 1.0 to 1.6 cm. At treatment distances of 1.8 cm and 2.0 cm, the relatively high dwell-times required at the end positions would have forced the second-position dwell-times to go negative in order to maintain dose uniformity among specification points. The compromise invoked by the algorithm in this situation is to drop both the second-position dwell times (setting them equal to zero) and the end-position specification points from the calculation, thereby reducing the number of unknowns (and equations) from four to three and accepting a slightly smaller end-position dose. This direct-solution method, which is very rapid and simple to implement on the computer, was initially proposed by Busch et al. in 1977.

In other treatment situations, exact answers may not be possible and a better method will be to seek dwell-times giving the best least-squares fit to the desired dose (Anderson, 1985). An example is the vaginal treatment plan depicted in **Fig. 5-14**, where the objective is a dose of 7 Gy in tissue on a contoured surface that is 0.5 cm deep in tissue in the upper portion of the treatment region and tapers to the applicator surface at the introitus. At the same time, it is desired to avoid hot spots (at the higher dose level) on the upper-half applicator surface. Specification points 1–7 control optimization at depth, while points 8–12 control surface uniformity. By appropriate weighting of the two groups of points in the calculation, a goodness-of-fit *balance* can be achieved between treatment dose at depth and surface dose uniformity. In this example, a standard deviation of 5.3 percent is realized among doses at treatment points versus 4.5 percent among doses at surface points.

GAMMA MED II DWELL TIMES FOR CYLINDRICAL DOSE CONTOURS
(by direct solution of linear equations)

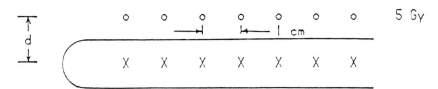

5 Gy

Treatment Distance d (cm)	Dwell Time (seconds)						
1.0	27	13	15	14	15	13	27
1.2	39	13	20	17	20	13	39
1.4	54	10	26	19	26	10	54
1.6	73	4	34	18	34	4	73
1.8	89	0	42	18	42	0	89
2.0	104	0	48	20	48	0	104

FIGURE 5-13

GAMMA MED VAGINAL APPLICATION, 2.3 cm DIA

MAG = 2.00

^{192}IR 10-CURIE SOURCE

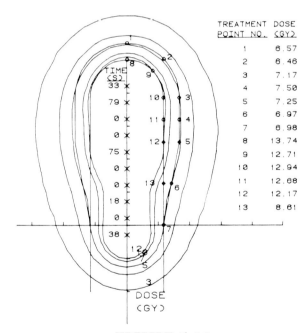

TREATMENT POINT NO.	DOSE (GY)
1	6.57
2	6.46
3	7.17
4	7.50
5	7.25
6	6.97
7	6.98
8	13.74
9	12.71
10	12.94
11	12.68
12	12.17
13	8.61

FIGURE 5-14

REFERENCES

1. Henschke, U. K. Afterloading applicator for radiation therapy of carcinoma of the uterus. *Radiology* 74:834, 1960.

2. Rosenstein, L. M. A simple computer program optimization of source loading in cervical applicators. *Br J Radiol* 50:119–122, 1977.

3. Mohan, R., Ding, I. Y., Toraskar, J., Chui, C., Anderson, L. L., and Nori, D. Computation of radiation dose distributions for shielded cervical applicators. *Int J Radiat Oncol Biol Phys* 11:823–830, 1985.

4. Cleaves, M. Radium: with a preliminary note on radium rays in the treatment of cancer. *Med Record* 64:601–606, 1903.

5. Cantril, S. T. *Radiation Therapy in the Management of Cancer of the Uterine Cervix.* Springfield, Ill.: C. C. Thomas, 1950, p. 189.

6. Tod, M. C., and Meredith, W. J. A dosage system for use in the treatment of cancer of the uterine cervix. *Br J Radiol* 11:809–824, 1938.

7. Meredith, W. J., ed. *Radium Dosage, The Manchester System.* Edinburgh: E & S Livingstone, 1967, p. 134.

8. Rosenstein, L. M. A simple computer program for optimization of source loading in cervical applicators. *Br J Radiol* 50:119–122, 1977.

9. Delclos, L., Fletcher, G. H., Sampiere, V., and Grant, W. H. Can the Fletcher gamma ray colpostat system be extrapolated to other systems? *Cancer* 41:970–979, 1978.

10. Anderson, L. L., Masterson, M. E., and Nori, D. Intracavitary radiation treatment planning and dose evaluation. In: Nori, D. (ed.): *Radiation Therapy of Gynecological Cancers.* New York: Alan R. Liss, 1987, pp. 51–71.

11. Masterson, M. E., Thomason, C., Hunt, M., Anderson, L. L., Eisenbarth, J., and Belanich, M. A comparative study of Henschke and Fletcher-Suit cervical applicators using Cs-137 (abstr.). *Int J Radiat Oncol Biol Phys* (Suppl. 1) 8:89, 1982.

12. Mohan, R., Ding, I. Y., Martel, M. K., Anderson, L. L., and Nori, D. Measurements of radiation dose distributions for shielded cervical applicators. *Int J Radiat Oncol Biol Phys* 11:861–868, 1985.

13. Drozdoff, V., Thomason, C., Anderson, L. L. 3D Cs-137 dose distribution for cervix applicator shielded ovoid (abstr.). *Med Phys* 10:536, 1983.

14. Mohan, R., Ding, I. Y., Toraskar, J., Chui, C., Anderson, L. L., and Nori, D. Computation of radiation dose distributions for shielded cervical applicators. *Int J Radiat Oncol Biol Phys* 11:823–830, 1985.

15. International Commission on Radiation Units and Measurement (ICRU). Dose and volume specification for reporting intracavitary therapy in gynecology. ICRU Report 38, International Commission on Radiation Units and Measurement, Bethesda, Maryland, 1985, p. 23.

16. Busch, M., Makosi, B., Schulz, U., and Saverwein, K. Das Essener Nachlade-Verfahren fur die intrakavitare Strahlentherapie. *Strahlentherapie* 153:581–588, 1977.

17. Anderson, L. L. Physical optimization of afterloading techniques. *Strahlentherapie* 161:264–269, 1985.

PART II

Clinical Applications of Brachytherapy

CHAPTER 6

Brachytherapy Techniques for Head and Neck Cancers

The majority of head and neck cancers, approximately 90 percent, are squamous-cell carcinomas and are largely related, epidemiologically, to alcohol and tobacco. The rest are carcinomas arising from the minor salivary glands and lymphomatous and sarcomatous tumors. Squamous-cell cancers generally progress by direct extension to surrounding tissues and then, by metastasizing, to the lymph nodes in the neck (**Fig. 6-1**). From the cervical lymph nodes, the metastases eventually spread to distant organs. The extent of the disease, for staging, can often be determined on clinical examination. For the more posteriorly situated lesions, however, an examination under anesthesia might be necessary (**Fig. 6-2**). In general, incidence rates for head and neck cancers have remained stable in the last 30 years. Reported overall survival rates improved somewhat from approximately 45 to 55 percent. The cure rates, however, range from 10 to 90 percent depending upon the pathologic type, histologic grade, tumor location, and tumor size. Most treatment failures occur within 2 years; locoregional recurrence is the rule and accounts for the majority of the deaths. Important advances have been made in the management of these cancers since 1950, with the most prominent occurring in surgery and radiation therapy and in the use of prosthodontics to reconstruct the facial area and help restore speech and mastication.

Brachytherapy is used as the definitive treatment of early superficial lesions of any size (T1–T4) with good expectation of local control, and in larger infiltrating lesions, as long as the size of the tumor is not more than 4 cm (small T2). In deeply invasive lesions (T3–T4) brachytherapy can be used either as 1) a "boost" after external irradiation to the primary site, 2) treatment after recurrence, or 3) after surgery whenever the margins of resection are suspected to be involved. Afterloading techniques are now used to the exclusion of the older radium techniques. Brachytherapy treatment planning utilizing modern imaging techniques, especially CT, is important in order to define the target volume in relation to the patient's anatomy as well as to display the calculated 3-D dose distribution.

Dental care must be initiated prior to the brachytherapy to avoid soft tissue or bone necrosis. Unrepairable teeth should be extracted. Fluoride treatments should be applied early and continue for the lifetime of the patient, especially if external therapy is integrated with brachytherapy.

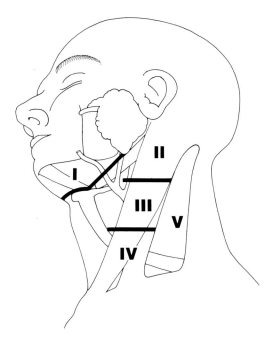

FIGURE 6-1

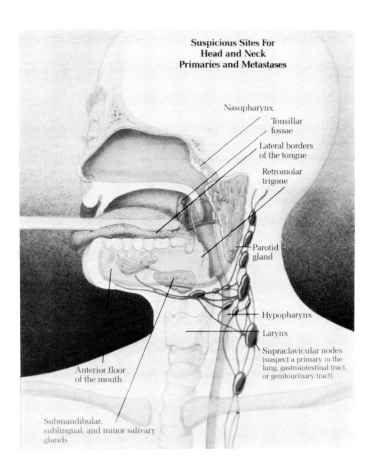

FIGURE 6-2

113

ORAL CAVITY

The *oral cavity* refers to the structures contained in the mouth anterior to the circumvalate papillae and anterior faucial pillars. It includes the lip, floor of the mouth, anterior two-thirds of the tongue, buccal mucosa, and hard palate.

Cancer of the Lip

This may be cured equally well with surgery or irradiation. Early lesions can be treated by interstitial brachytherapy alone with excellent cosmetic results. Large lesions, with the exception of mandibular extension, may be treated by integrated external beam and brachytherapy. In addition, advanced lesions and/or recurrent lesions should have elective neck node dissection or neck irradiation.

The Recommended Interstitial Brachytherapy Technique. This is the basic temporary Ir-192 technique, performed either under local anesthesia for small lesions or general anesthesia for large lesions (**Fig. 6-3**). Small superficial lesions require only a single plane, but larger lesions require a two-plane implant, containing horizontally placed parallel plastic tubes. In many European centers a hypodermic needle technique is preferred over the plastic tube technique.

The Target Volume. This includes the tumor and a 0.5-cm margin beyond the palpable tumor border in all directions; larger lesions require a 1-cm margin.

The Target Dose. This is 6000 cGy for small lesions, and a higher total dose of 7000 to 7500 cGy for larger lesions (4500 to 5000 cGy with external beam and 2500 cGy by brachytherapy).

Cancer of the Floor of the Mouth

The majority of these lesions begin within the anterior midline floor of the mouth (**Fig. 6-4,** left); lesions of the lateral floor are rare. The first nodes involved are the submandibular and the subdigastric; lesions crossing the midline have a high risk of bilateral spread.

Extension towards the gingiva and the periosteum of the mandible occurs early, but mandible invasion is usually a late manifestation.

Recommended Interstitial Brachytherapy Technique. The loop temporary implant IR-192 technique is recommended. Small lesions usually require a two-loop implant; larger lesions require a multiloop implant. The guide gutter technique can be substituted for the plastic tube technique.

The Target Volume. Includes the tumor volume and 1-cm margin around it.

The Target Dose. This is 6000 cGy for small lesions (Fig. 6-4, right). Patients with larger lesions or with cervical node metastases should receive a brachytherapy boost dose of 2500 cGy 2 to 3 weeks after the completion of 5000 cGy external radiation. An intense, but localized mucositis appears 8 to 10 days after completion of implantation (**Fig. 6-5,** left). The same patient 3 years after treatment, with no evidence of disease (Fig. 6-5 right).

114

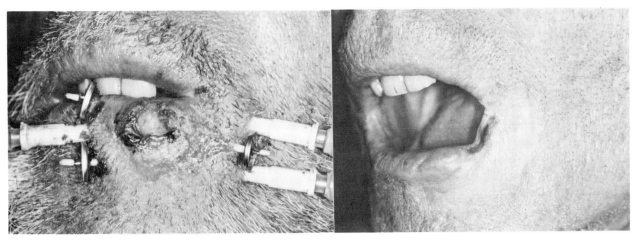

FIGURE 6-3

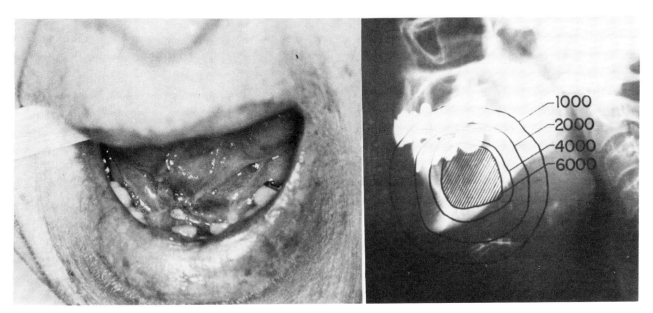

FIGURE 6-4

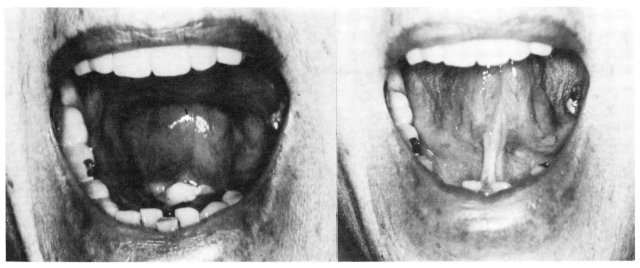

FIGURE 6-5

Cancer of the Anterior Two-Thirds of the Tongue

Nearly all cancers of the oral tongue occur on the lateral surfaces of the tongue and only rarely on the dorsum (**Fig. 6-6**). The first echelon of neck node spread is in the subdigastric and submandibular nodes. Thirty-five percent of patients with oral cancer have clinically positive nodes (5 percent bilateral). Surgery and irradiation produce similar cure rates. Treatment decisions, therefore, are based on anticipated functional loss, management of the neck, and patient preference. The ability to control the primary tumor by irradiation is enhanced by giving all or most of the dose by brachytherapy. Definitive interstitial brachytherapy is the preferable choice for larger T1–T2 lesions in order to preserve speech and swallowing. External beam irradiation of the neck is recommended for all primary anterior tongue lesions larger than 1 cm in diameter.

Brachytherapy Technique. The loop afterloading temporary Ir-192 technique is recommended. Retracting the tongue anteriorly and to the contralateral side of the mouth gives a better view of the tumor. The first two loops are positioned in the anterior and posterior margins of the tumor (**Fig. 6-7**A–C). Subsequent loops, if necessary, are implanted between them at equal distances, usually 1.2 to 1.5 cm (Fig. 6-7D).

The guide gutter technique is favored in many European centers for small lesions, but it requires cumbersome radiation protection measures (mobile lead screens) to decrease radiation exposure. Although the brachytherapy procedure can be done under local or regional (bilateral mandibular) anesthesia with the patient sitting upright in a dental chair, we favor general anesthesia, especially for larger lesions because it allows an unhurried and more accurate implementation of the procedure.

The Target Volume. Includes the tumor (in boost therapy the original extent of the tumor) and 1-cm margin.

The Target Dose. This is 6500 to 7000 cGy when brachytherapy is used alone or 3000 to 3500 cGy as a boost dose following 4500 to 5000 cGy by external beam.

Orthogonal x-rays are taken with dummy sources to determine the source location (Fig. 6-7E) and to allow computerized dose calculations. An example of a 3-D target dose calculation is shown in Fig. 6-7F.

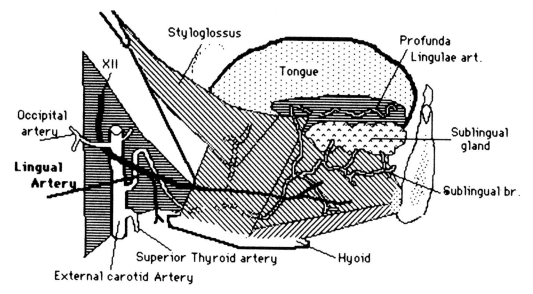

FIGURE 6-6

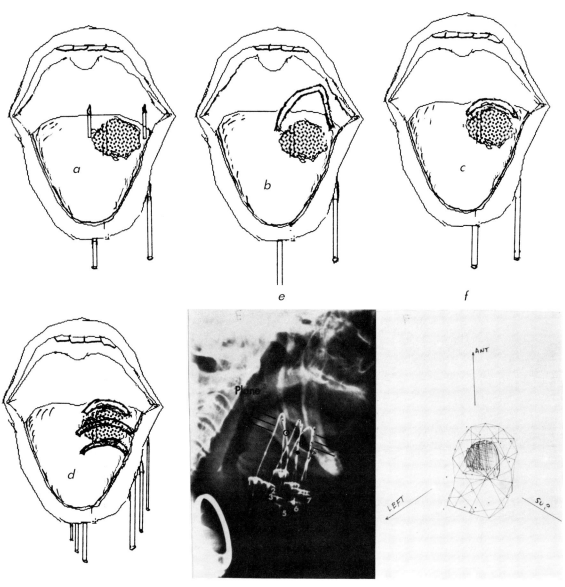

FIGURE 6-7

Cancer of the Buccal Mucosa

Almost all of the squamous cell carcinomas of the buccal mucosa originate on the mucous membrane covering the inner surface of the cheeks. Only advanced larger lesions penetrate the underlying muscles and eventually the skin. The lymphatic spread is first to the submandibular and subdigastric nodes. Interstitial brachytherapy alone is indicated for small to moderate size lesions with no extension to the gingivobuccal sulcus or onto bone. A lead block placed in the mouth will help decrease radiation to other normal structures within the oral cavity.

Brachytherapy Interstitial Technique. Lesions of the buccal mucosa are implanted percutaneously under general anesthesia, using either the basic temporary implant technique (**Fig. 6-8**: left-schematic drawing; right-actual procedure) or the sealed-end temporary implant technique (**Fig. 6-9**: left-actual procedure; right-schematic drawing). A single plane implant is used for superficial lesions; a two-plane implant is preferable for deeply invasive disease. In the latter arrangement, it is advisable to direct each plane's lines in a different direction, i.e., perpendicular to each other, to facilitate their identification in the post-implantation localization films. Planes must be separated by a 1.2 to 1.5-cm distance. A loop implant technique or guide gutter might be substituted, in small lesions, for the preceding techniques.

The Target Volume. Includes the tumor volume and a 1-cm margin of normal tissue around the tumor.

The Target Dose. Recommended for early lesions (T1 and early T2) without involvement of the gingiva is 6500 cGy; for larger lesions in which elective irradiation of the first nodal station is indicated, a boost dose of 2500 to 3000 cGy is given after 4500 to 5000 cGy external beam.

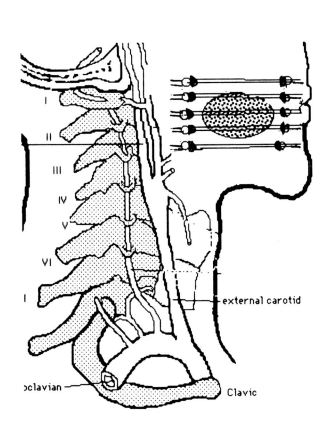

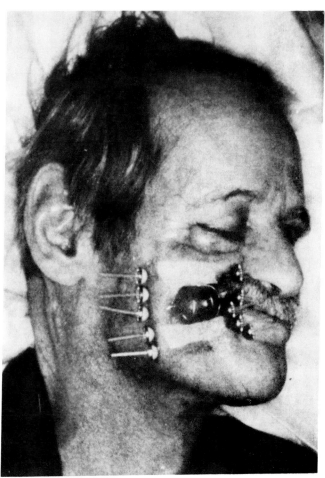

external carotid

Clavic

oclavian

FIGURE 6-8

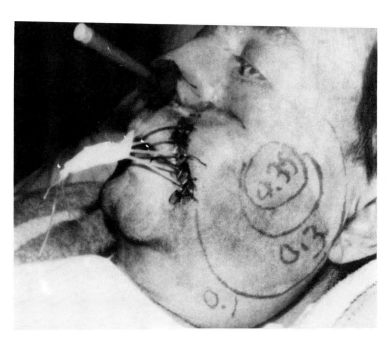

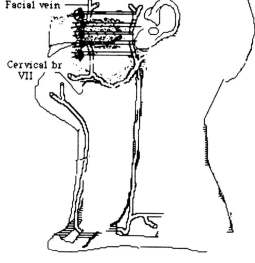

Facial vein

Cervical br VII

FIGURE 6-9

Cancer of the Hard Palate

Primary squamous cell carcinoma in this location is uncommon. Most of the lesions in this site are minor salivary gland tumors (**Fig. 6-10**: left—before radiation; right—4 months after radiation with a customized applicator).

Brachytherapy Technique. The usual indication for brachytherapy is an early superficial lesion extensively involving the hard palate, with little or no bone involvement. These lesions are best treated by customized intraoral surface applicators (**Fig. 6-11**). Manual afterloading with Ir-192 or I-125 seeds is performed. The latter affords the advantage of easy shielding of the neighboring normal tissue. High dose rate remote afterloading with Ir-192 is an alternative option allowing treatment on an outpatient basis.

Target Volume. Includes the visible lesion plus a 1-cm margin around it.

Target Dose. A dose of 6500 to 7000 cGy is given with low dose rate conventional Ir-192 or I-125 manual afterloading.

If remote afterloading with high intensity Ir-192 sources is used, a total dose of 3600 to 4200 cGy is given in 6–7 fractions, not exceeding 600 cGy per application/week (**Fig. 6-12**).

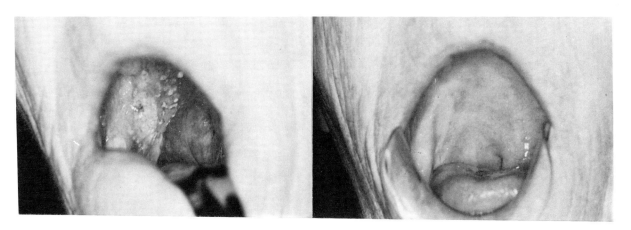

FIGURE 6-10

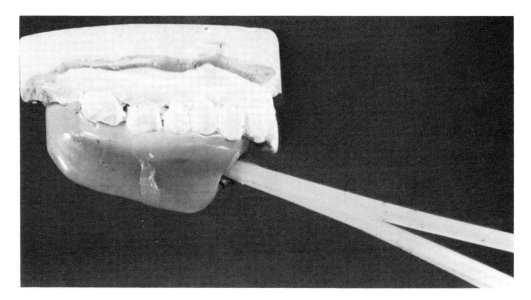

FIGURE 6-11

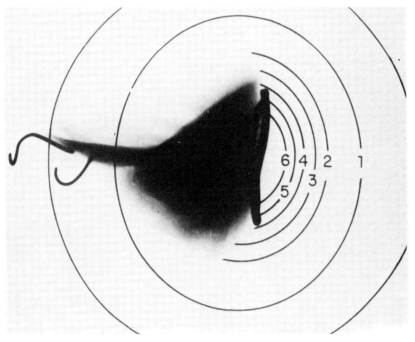

FIGURE 6-12

OROPHARYNX

The *oropharynx* includes the base of the tongue, the tonsillar fossa and tonsillar pillars, the soft palate, and the posterior and lateral pharyngeal wall from the level of the soft palate to the level of the hyoid bone (**Fig. 6-13**, anterior and lateral view). Tumors in these locations are usually treated by external irradiation that encompasses the primary lesion and both sides of the neck. Brachytherapy is recommended as a *boost* therapy following a moderate dose of external radiation. Interstitial brachytherapy should be performed under general anesthesia to allow for better exposure of the lesion. A preliminary tracheostomy is desirable in these patients, in contrast to patients with more anteriorly located lesions, to avoid respiratory obstruction caused by edema or hemorrhage occurring during or immediately after the procedure. Feeding by a nasal tube, adequate sedation, and pain medication are recommended during the period that the implant is in place.

Cancer of the Base of the Tongue

Tumors of the base of the tongue tend to remain localized, except if they begin at the peripheral margin of the tongue; in the latter instance they may invade either the glossotonsillar sulcus or spread along the mucosa to the lingual surface of the epiglottis, the pharyngoepiglottic fold and then the lateral pharyngeal wall. The first echelon of nodal spread is in the subdigastric nodes, and then to midjugular and lower jugular. The posterior cervical nodes are often involved. Interstitial brachytherapy is used as a boost therapy in small to moderate size, discrete lesions located preferably in the anteriolateral base of the tongue.

Recommended Brachytherapy Technique. This is the loop temporary Ir-192 implantation (**Fig. 6-14**). Note the use of an intraoral lead shield for protecting the soft and hard palate in this figure. It can be easily constructed to fit the individual patient and provides adequate protection of the surrounding normal tissue because of the relatively low energy of Ir-192. The loop temporary implant technique has been described previously in details in Chap. 3.

The Target Volume. This includes the original extent of the tumor and a 1-cm margin around the tumor.

The Target Dose. Consists of 5000 cGy given by external beam and an interstitial boost of 2500 to 3000 cGy.

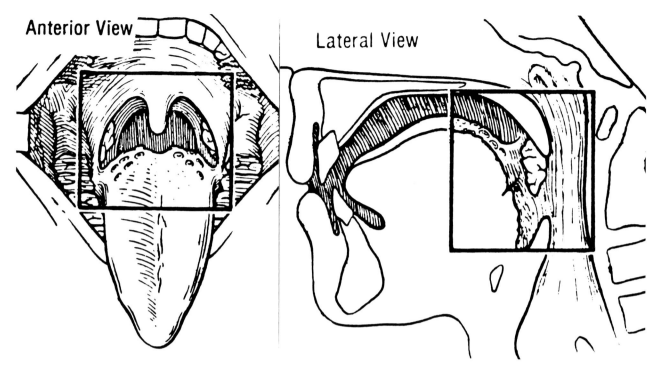

Anterior View

Lateral View

FIGURE 6-13

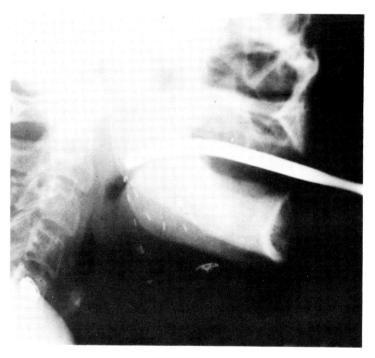

FIGURE 6-14

MODIFICATIONS OF LOOP TECHNIQUE

Soon after the development of the loop technique, it became evident that its use was technically more difficult, and many radiotherapists had difficulties in executing the *loop* and, therefore, in performing a satisfactory implant in the base of the tongue. Furthermore, at times, a nylon tube may kink at its looping portion and it can no longer be negotiated by the ribbon containing the radioactive seeds.

That led to the development of several modifications of the loop technique, used at Memorial Sloan Kettering Cancer Center, which will be described in the next few pages.

Loop Wire Technique (Hilaris–Henschke)

This modification of the loop technique allows much of the work to be done outside the mouth while retaining the afterloading principle.

An example of this technique will be illustrated in its application to a localized lesion of the base of the tongue (**Fig. 6-15A**).

A preliminary tracheostomy is recommended in all base of the tongue implants. The procedure is performed under general anesthesia to allow an unhurried inspection of the tumor and execution of the procedure. The patient's head is well extended.

With the brachytherapist's index finger in the patient's mouth, a standard stainless-steel implantation needle is inserted through the submandibular region, in a posterior and superior direction and pushed toward the tumor in the base of the tongue (Fig. 6-15B).

The operator always works with a pair of needles, as in the standard loop technique. Each needle is pushed into the mouth until it pierces the mucosa of the base of the tongue (Fig. 6-15C, internal view).

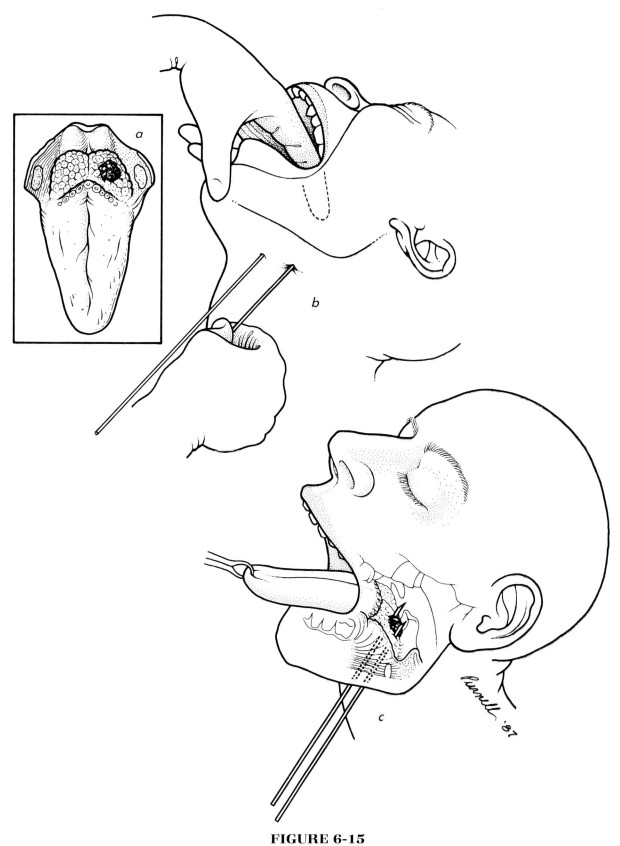

FIGURE 6-15

A surgical medium-size wire, readily available in all operating rooms, is introduced through the proximal (neck) end of needle number 1, and it is advanced through the oral cavity, allowing 15 to 20 cm length of wire to be exposed outside of the mouth (Fig. 6-15D).

The next step is to clamp the wire at the proximal (neck) tip of the needle (Fig. 6-15E).

Afterloading nylon tubes are prepared by cutting off the thin portion (leader), on either side of the tube. One afterloading catheter is slipped over the distal (oral) end of the wire and advanced until it reaches the tip of the needle (Fig. 6-15F).

The distal (oral) end of the wire is clamped at the tip of the catheter (Fig. 6-15G).

The needle is now slowly withdrawn completely from the neck, thereby pulling the catheter tip into the base of the tongue and out through the neck (Fig. 6-15H).

At this point the clamp is removed from the wire at the distal (oral) tip of catheter (Fig. 6-15I).

The wire is then completely withdrawn from the entire length of the catheter (Fig. 6-15J).

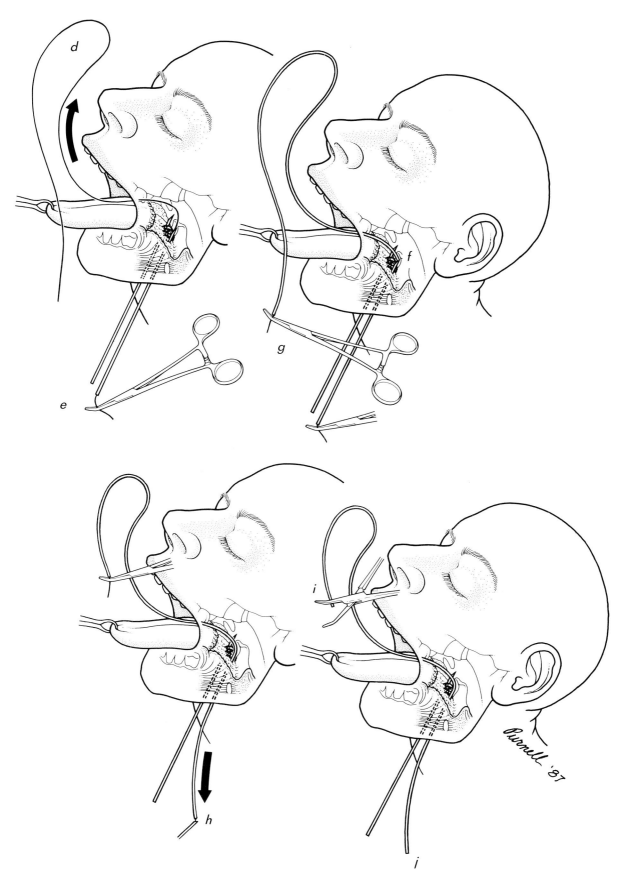

FIGURE 6-15 (Continued)

The next step is essentially similar to the previous one. A wire is introduced into the proximal (neck) end of needle number 2 (Fig. 6-15K).

This wire is advanced into and through the oral cavity to the distal (oral) tip of nylon catheter, into which the wire is inserted (Fig. 6-15L).

The wire is slowly advanced until it emerges from the distal (neck) tip of the plastic catheter and is clamped (Fig. 6-15M).

The wire is now pulled (Fig. 6-15N) so that it draws the distal (oral) tip of the catheter into apposition to that of the needle (Fig. 6-15L–O; P).

The wire is clamped at the distal (neck) tip of the needle (Fig. 6-15Q).

The needle is slowly withdrawn completely from the neck, pulling with it the catheter tip into the base of the tongue and out through the neck (Fig. 6-15R).

At this point the brachytherapist puts his index finger in loop of plastic catheter to prevent kinking as loop size is decreased (Fig. 6-15S).

The catheter is pulled until it is apposed to surface of tongue (Fig. 6-15T).

The final illustration is a view of root of tongue after placement of three afterloading catheters at the tumor site (Fig. 6-15U).

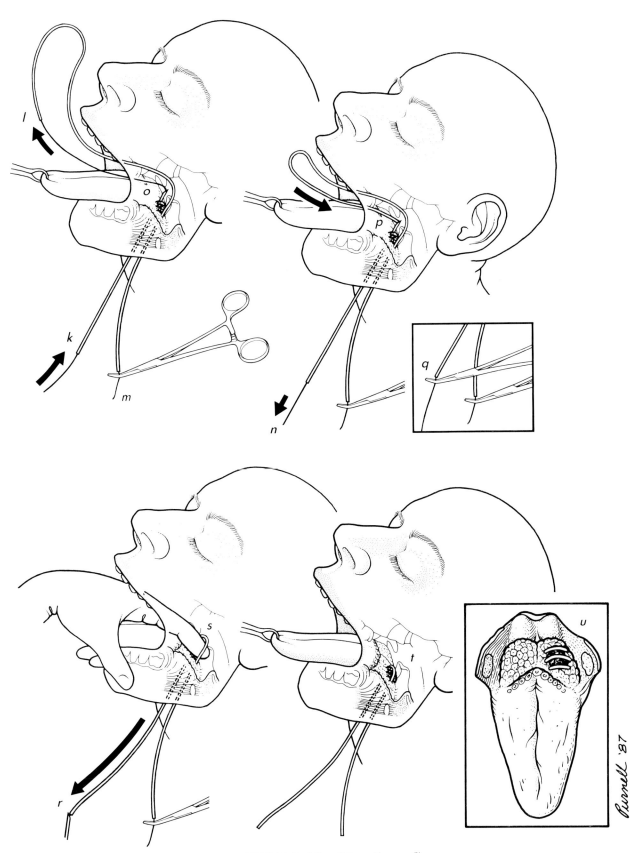

FIGURE 6-15 (Continued)

Nonlooping Technique (Vikram–Hilaris Technique)

This technique is another modification of the loop technique for the implantation of the base of the tongue. The procedure is performed after a preliminary tracheostomy and under general anesthesia. It is an alternative option to the loop technique when there is lack of space for maneuvering inside the mouth.

With the operator's index finger in the mouth and the patient's head well extended, stainless-steel needles are introduced through the submandibular region into the tongue until their tip pierces the mucosa of the base of the tongue (**Fig. 6-16**, left).

A plastic afterloading catheter with the one end sealed is then introduced through each needle into the pharynx and brought outside the mouth. Their closed ends (2 to 3 mm from the tip) are sutured to a horizontal *crossing* plastic catheter (Fig. 6-16, right).

The needles are then withdrawn from the neck and the whole plane of the plastic catheters is brought into position until the crossing catheter lies on the dorsum of the tongue (**Fig. 6-17**, left). The plastic catheters are secured on the skin as usual by means of a plastic hemisphere and a metal button (Fig. 6-17, right). The crossing catheter may be brought out through the mouth and be secured on the cheek.

As many needles as are necessary can be introduced in a similar manner (**Fig. 6-18**, left).

After the localization and dosimetric studies are completed, the catheters are afterloaded with Ir-192 seeds (Fig. 6-18, right).

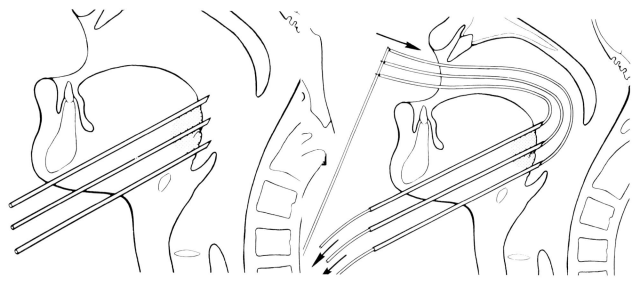

FIGURE 6-16

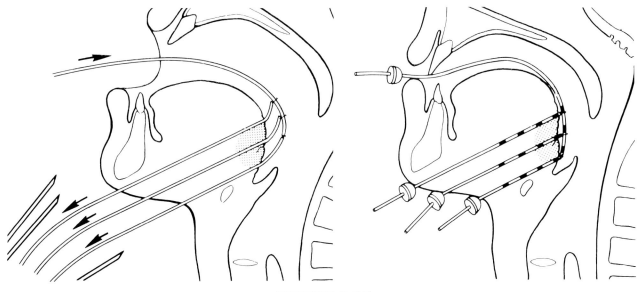

FIGURE 6-17

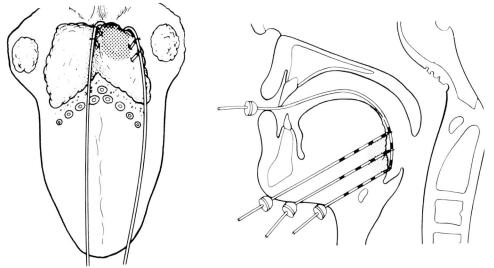

FIGURE 6-18

Cancer of the Tonsillar Region

The tonsillar region includes the anterior and posterior tonsillar pillars and the tonsillar fossa. Almost all malignant lesions arising in this location are squamous cell carcinomas. These lesions have a very high incidence of metastases in the ipsilateral cervical lymph nodes; therefore, the neck should always be irradiated by external beam. The risk for contralateral lymph node metastases is small, unless there is tumor extension to the tongue, soft palate close to the midline, or clinically positive nodes in the ipsilateral neck. Interstitial brachytherapy alone can be considered for the occasional very small superficial lesion or as a boost for locally advanced lesions in combination with external therapy. Normal tissue sequellae are less with this approach than with external beam alone.

Recommended Interstitial Brachytherapy Technique. The recommended technique is the loop Ir-192 temporary implantation. Two or more sagittally oriented loops are used, with a separation of 1.2 to 1.5 cm (**Fig. 6-19**).

The Target Volume. Includes the palpable lesion and a 1-cm margin around it.

The Target Dose. This dose by the implant is 2500 to 3000 cGy given after an external beam dose of 4500 to 5000 cGy.

Cancer of the Soft Palate and Pharyngeal Wall

Tumors in these locations are almost exclusively in the oral site of the palate or the hypopharyngeal walls. The incidence of positive nodes increases with T stage (8 to 66 percent).

Recommended Interstitial Technique. The recommended technique is the basic permanent implantation or the absorbable Vicryl suture technique described previously.

Target Volume. The target volume includes the palpable or visible lesion and a 1-cm margin around it.

Target Dose. For an I-125 permanent implant, the target dose ranges from 16,000 to 30,000 cGy.

A technique recently described by Son is illustrated in **Fig. 6-20**. The lower hypopharynx is approached by keeping the patient's neck hyperextended while the tongue is retracted upward.

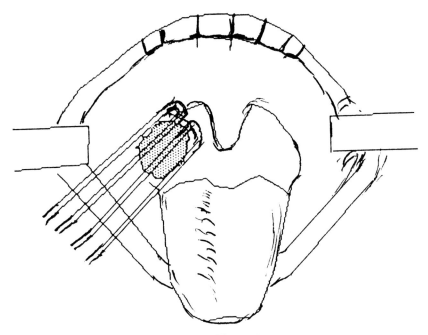

FIGURE 6-19

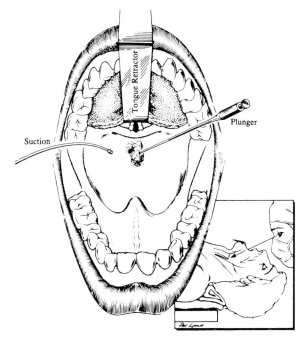

FIGURE 6-20

OTHER UNUSUAL LOCATIONS

Other unusual locations in which brachytherapy can be applied include the nasopharyngeal cavity, the nasal cavity, and the maxillary sinuses.

Cancer of the Nasopharynx

This often spreads beyond the confines of the nasopharyngeal cavity to the base of the skull superiorly, to the nasal cavity anteriorly, to the pterygo-maxillary space laterally, and to the oropharynx inferiorly. The first echelon of lymph nodes involved is the retropharyngeal and upper cervical groups. Thus, external beam therapy is used to treat both the primary site and the neck. Brachytherapy is used either for the treatment of recurrent nasopharyngeal carcinoma or to administer a boost dose to the primary tumor at the conclusion of external beam therapy in previously untreated patients. CT scanning with both transverse and coronal views is a most valuable study to determine the extent of the tumor, as well as for treatment planning. The choice of interstitial versus intracavitary technique depends on the extent of the residual or recurrent lesion and on its location within the nasopharyngeal cavity.

Intracavitary Technique. The intracavitary technique is recommended for superficial lesions that diffusely involve the nasopharyngeal cavity, but not the bone. A variety of nasopharyngeal applicators has been used. A detailed description is beyond the scope of this book. We will illustrate the two approaches we have personally utilized for several years.

TRANSNASAL APPROACH. The first step of this technique consists of the insertion of the unloaded applicator, which is carried out under local anesthesia. The applicator is made of an acrylic plastic sphere (3.0 cm, 2.5 cm, and 2.0 cm in diameter) connected to two nylon tubes. To insert the applicator in the nasopharyngeal cavity, two small rubber catheters are first introduced through the nose and brought through the mouth. The oral end of each catheter is then connected to one of the nylon tubes of the applicator. The rubber catheters and the nylon tubes are then pulled back through the nose and the plastic sphere is pushed at the same time with a finger behind the uvula until it lies in the nasopharyngeal cavity (**Fig. 6-21**, left).

After localization films have confirmed the proper positioning of the application (Fig. 6-21, middle) the radioactive sources are afterloaded into the applicator either manually (Fig. 6-21, right) or by remote control.

Various other custom made applicators can be used (**Fig. 6-22**, left). Computerized isodose contours may be displayed by superimposing them to the orthogonal radiographs (Fig. 6-22, right).

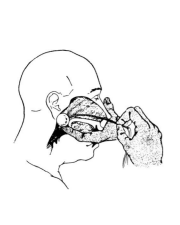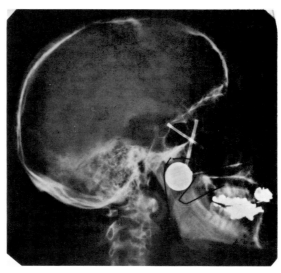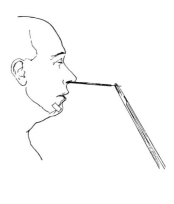

FIGURE 6-21

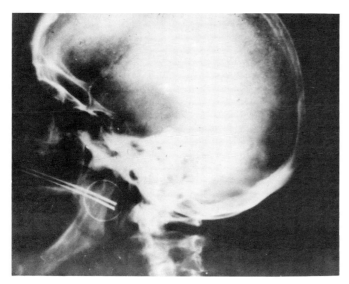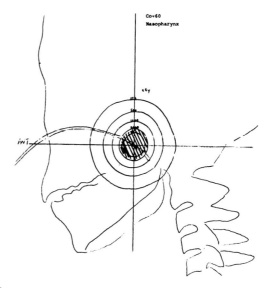

FIGURE 6-22

TRANSORAL APPROACH. This is performed using the remote afterloading high dose rate technique. The patient sits on a dental chair equipped with a head-support.

A nasopharyngeal kit is commercially available and contains the following items:

5 curved tubes with various curves
5 acrylic plastic locking devices with knurled locking screw
various hemispherical "balls" (1.5, 2.0, and 2.5 cm in diameter)
1 McKesson disposable mouthpiece, adult size
1 short inflatable cuff with pilot balloon (5 cc)
(The last two items are replaced after each use)

The procedure is performed under local anesthesia. It is essential that the uvula, oropharynx and nasopharynx are well anesthetized in addition to the oral mucosa. The length of the nasopharyngeal cavity and the curvature necessary to enter it through the mouth are measured using a flexible sound, such as the one used for probing the uterine cavity.

The metal tube size and curvature most appropriate for the individual patient is selected. An appropriate size "ball" (**Fig. 6-23**) or, if preferred, a short inflatable cuff with a pilot balloon (**Fig. 6-24**) is attached to the tip of the tube. The balloon is tested with air to make sure that it does not leak. The McKesson disposable mouthpiece is adjusted to the proper distance so it fits between the upper and lower teeth. The assembled applicator is then ready for insertion. The applicator is slightly rotated and pushed behind the uvula. It is then rotated and positioned in the middle of the nasopharynx. The patient is instructed to bite lightly on the mouthpiece. The balloon is inflated with 10 to 20 cc of air and the catheter is clamped to retain the air.

The position of the applicator is checked with a localization film (**Fig. 6-25**, left). The applicator is then connected to the remote afterloading unit and the treatment is begun (Fig. 6-25, right).

Target Dose. If a conventional low dose rate is used, a boost dose of 2500 to 3000 cGy is given at 0.5 cm from the surface of the applicator following 5000 cGy external beam. If a high dose rate is utilized, a boost dose of 1500 to 2000 cGy is delivered in 3 to 4 weekly fractions of 500 cGy each.

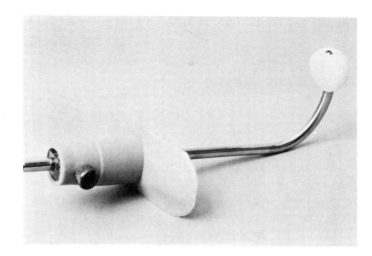

FIGURE 6-23

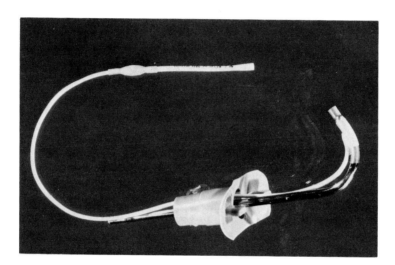

FIGURE 6-24

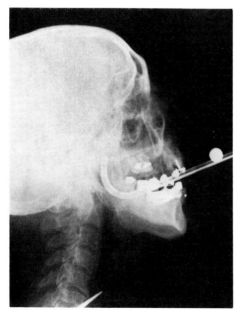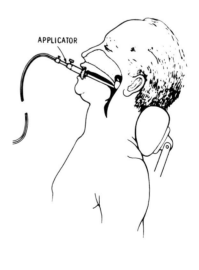

APPLICATOR

FIGURE 6-25

Interstitial Technique This is recommended for patients with localized persistent or recurrent tumor without bone extension following external beam radiation.

Transpalatal Approach This is used for lesions (> 0.5 cm) located in the posterior wall or lateral walls of the nasopharynx. The procedure is performed under general anesthesia. A transverse mucosal incision is made at the junction of the hard and soft palate. A large segment of the hard palate is removed, exposing the nasopharynx, as first described by Wilson. This defect in the hard palate permits a thorough inspection of the nasopharynx during the implantation and allows the insertion of the radioactive sources in and around the tumor (**Fig. 6-26**, left). The defect is subsequently closed by a palatal plate similar to an upper dental plate. Localization films are used to determine and evaluate the dose distribution (Fig. 6-26, right).

Transnasal Approach (Vikram's Technique This approach is recommended for lesions in the posterior wall or the roof of the nasopharynx. The procedure is performed under general anesthesia, with the patient in supine position and the head slightly elevated. The uvula is retracted forward with a loop retractor and the nasopharynx is visualized through the mouth, using a fiberoptic nasopharyngoscope (**Fig. 6-27**, left). After satisfactory visualization of the area of concern, radioactive I-125 seeds are introduced through the nasal passages into the nasopharynx and inserted into the tumor submucosally using the basic permanent implantation technique (Fig. 6-27, right). Blood loss during the procedure is minimal. Most patients are able to go home the same day or next morning.

Target Volume. In either of the preceding approaches, the target volume includes the visualized tumor plus a 0.5 to 1-cm margin around it.

Target Dose. Varies from 16,000 to 32,000 cGy depending on the average dimension of the lesion. It is calculated using the New York System of dosimetry.

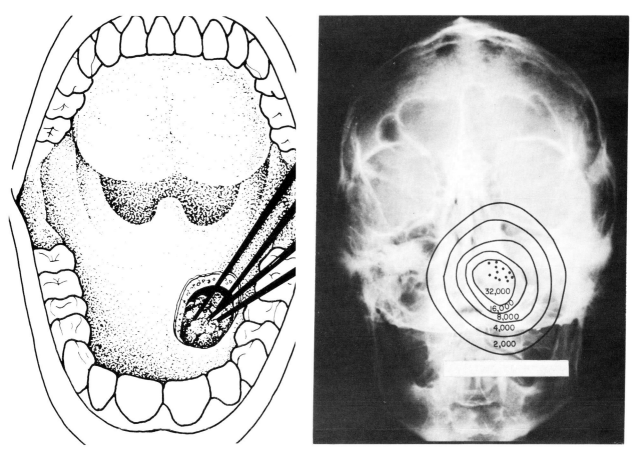

FIGURE 6-26

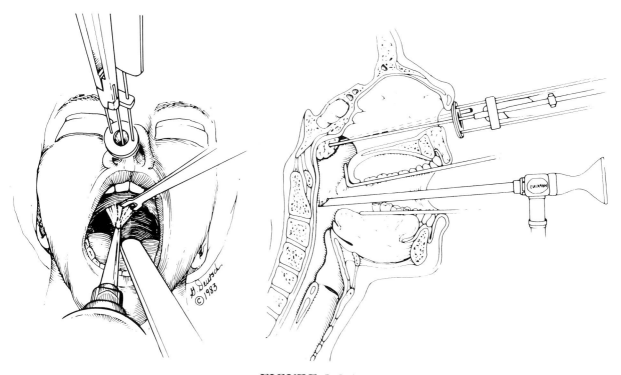

FIGURE 6-27

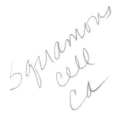
Squamous cell Ca

NECK NODE METASTASES

Since its introduction more than 100 years ago, radical neck dissection has been the treatment of choice for most resectable neck node metastases from squamous cell carcinoma of the head and neck region. Neck irradiation using photon or electron beams is an alternative option utilized for certain head and neck tumors. Interstitial brachytherapy is usually reserved for patients with persisting disease after external beam or surgical resection and for recurrent disease after unsuccessful surgery or radiation.

Temporary Afterloading Brachytherapy Technique

The basic implantation technique is utilized in the curative management of massive neck metastases or recurrences, or intraoperatively following an incomplete neck dissection. This technique is more elaborate requiring in most cases general anesthesia and hospitalization.

In most institutions, the implant is being done as a separate procedure. A single- or two-plane implant, using flexible plastic catheters, is usually satisfactory. When large lesions are to be treated, perpendicular source lines in alternate planes are preferred (**Fig. 6-28**, left). Although excellent local control is expected, severe late fibrosis is not uncommon (Fig. 6-28, right). Bulkier tumors may require an even larger implant (**Fig. 6-29**, left). Orthogonal localization x-rays are taken as usual prior to afterloading (Fig. 6-29, right).

Tumor bed (intraoperative) temporary Ir-192 implants are being recommended as a supplement or boost to external radiation in selected patients with residual tumor or close margins after neck dissection.

Target Volume.   Determined by palpation, visual inspection, and, in larger nodes, by CT scans. It includes the tumor (nodes) plus an adequate margin, which is decided on an individual basis.

Target Dose.   For temporary implants the dose is 6000 to 6500 cGy in 5 to 7 days, calculated at least 0.5 cm from the plane of the implant. If a previous external beam in the range of 5000 cGy has been used, a boost dose of 2500 to 3000 cGy is given.

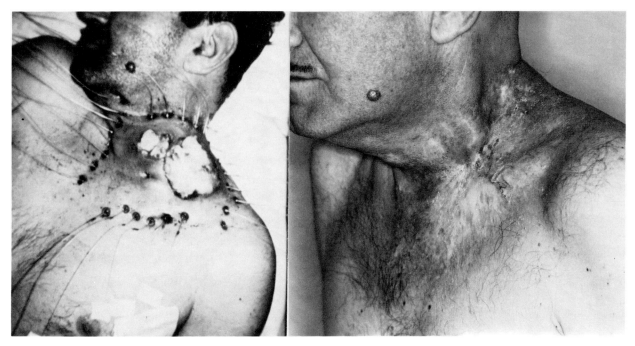

FIGURE 6-28

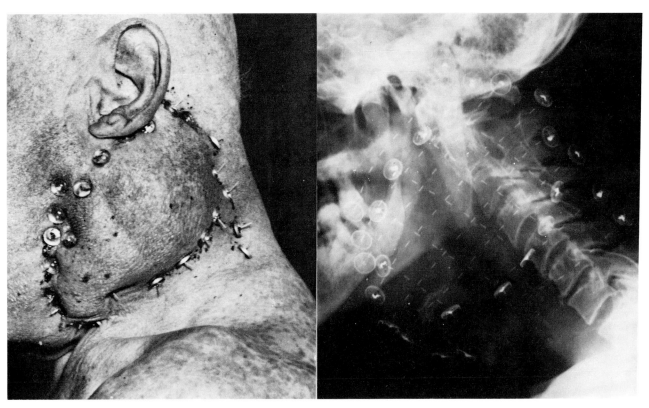

FIGURE 6-29

Permanent Afterloading Brachytherapy Technique

Permanent implants are used for the treatment of small or moderate size lymph nodes that cannot be resected or for tumor bed implantation (at the completion of neck dissection prior to myocutaneous flap coverage) when the surgical margin of resection is suspected to be involved by the tumor.

The basic permanent implantation technique or the I-125 Vicryl suture technique are recommended. Most of the palliative permanent implants can be done on an outpatient basis under local anesthesia. Small nodes can be treated effectively by a single-or two-plane implant; larger nodes require a volume implant. (**Fig. 6-30**, right). Tumor regression occurs within a fairly rapid time after implantation, achieving quick palliation (Fig. 6-30, left).

For permanent I-125 implants a minimum dose of 16,000 cGy is administered using the New York System of dosimetry.

Dosimetry for permanent and temporary implants should be based on orthogonal films taken with dummy sources, a lead wire on the skin surface overlying the implanted region, and a lead wire outlining the tumor volume (**Fig. 6-31**, left). Computerized calculations can be overlaid to display the dose distribution (Fig. 6-31, right). CT scans, if available, can be used to determine the tumor extent and to display the dose distribution.

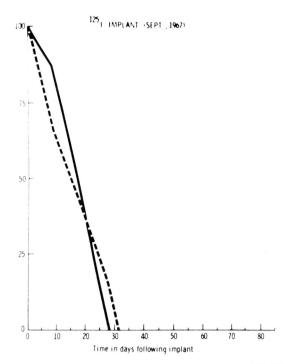

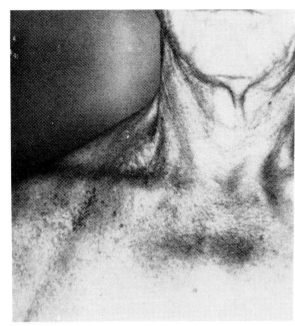

FIGURE 6-30

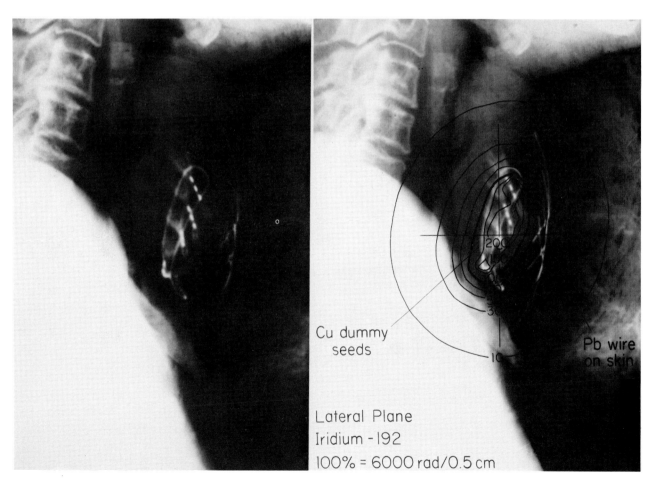

Cu dummy
seeds

Pb wire
on skin

Lateral Plane
Iridium -192
100% = 6000 rad/0.5 cm

FIGURE 6-31

143

RESULTS

Extensive experience with interstitial brachytherapy has been accumulated in several European and American centers. **Table 6-1** summarizes some of this experience.

Thus, at the Institute Gustave-Roussy in Paris, France, 51 patients with cancer of the floor of the mouth, stages T1 and T2, treated by brachytherapy achieved a 5-year actuarial survival of 72 percent.

At the same center, 119 patients with cancer of the mobile tongue, stages T1 and T2, that were managed mainly with the gutter guide technique had a 5-year actuarial survival of 50 percent.

The Creteil experience, in France, with epidermoid cancer of the tonsil in 33 patients that were treated by a combination of external beam and brachytherapy is equally good. The actuarial 5-year disease-free survival was 76 percent for all patients, and 80 percent for patients with negative nodes.

Vikram reported the Memorial experience with a combination of external beam and a brachytherapy boost in cancer of the base of the tongue. In the first 20 patients, no locoregional failures were observed during the period of follow-up, which ranged from 1 to 5 years.

Vtyurin et al. have reported the experience in the Soviet Union with Cf-257 in the treatment of 47 patients with cancer of the base of the tongue. The local control was 77 percent with a minimum follow-up of 1 year.

In cancer of the lip interstitial brachytherapy has demonstrated 5-year disease-free survival of more than 90-percent (Pigneux et al.)

The Stanford experience with I-125 permanent Vicryl suture brachytherapy was reported by Martinez et al. Local control was 79 percent in 14 previously untreated patients and 59 percent in 34 previously treated patients.

TABLE 6-1. Brachytherapy Results in Early Lesions

Author	Site	# Pts	5-Yr Survival (%)
Haie et al.	Floor of mouth	61	72
Haie et al.	Oral tongue	155	50
Mazeron	Tonsil	33	76
Pigneux et al.	Lip	91	94
Baillet et al.	Base of tongue	24	54
Pernot et al.	Buccal mucosa	211	64 (3 yr)

REFERENCES

1. Gerbaulet, A., Chassagne, D., Hayem, M., and Vandenbrouck, C. Carcinoma of the lip. A series of 335 cases. *J Radiol Electrol Med Nucl* 59:603–610, 1978.

2. Pigneux, J., Richaud, P. M., and Lagarde, C. The place of interstitial therapy using 192 iridium in the management of carcinoma of the lip. *Cancer* 43:1073–1077, 1979.

3. Petrovien, Z., Kuisk, H., Tobochnik, N., Hittle, R. E., Barton, R., and Jose, L. Carcinoma of the lip. *Arch Otolaryngol* 105:187–191, 1979.

4. Delclos, L. Interstitial irradiation techniques. In: *Technological Basis of Radiation Therapy: Practical Clinical Applications*, Levitt, S. H., and Tapley, N. D. (eds.). Philadelphia: Lea and Febiger, 1984, pp. 55–100.

5. Haie, C., Chassagne, D., and Gerbaulet, A. Results of brachytherapy in the management of oral cavity cancer (abstr.). *Endocuriether/Hyperthermia Oncol* 2:60, 1986.

6. Baillet, F., Decroix, Y., Mazeron, J. J.: Oral tongue. In: *Modern Brachytherapy*, Pierquin, B., Wilson, J. F., and Chassagne, D. (eds.). Paris; Masson, 1987, Chap. 12, pp. 107–118.

7. Mazeron, J. J., Calitchi, E., Martin, M., Maylin, C., Le Bourgeois, J. P., Lobo, P., Baillet, F., and Pierquin, B. Analysis of local failures after treatment with curietherapy using iridium-192 for squamous cell carcinoma of the mobile tongue. *J Eur Radiother* 3:139–144, 1982.

8. Pernot, M., and Gerbaulet, A. Buccal mucosa. In: *Modern Brachytherapy*. Pierquin, B., Wilson, J. F., and Chassagne, D. (eds.). Paris: Masson, 1978, Chap. 6, pp. 101–106.

9. Goffinet, D. R., Martinez, A., Palos, B., Fee, W., and Bagshaw, M. A. A method of interstitial tonsillo-palatine implants. *Int J Radiat Oncol Biol Phys* 2:155–162, 1977.

10. Vikram, B., and Hilaris, B. S. A non-looping afterloading technique for interstitial implants of the base of the tongue. *Int J Radiat Oncology Biol Phys* 7:419–422, 1981.

11. Vikram, B., Strong, E. W., Shah, J. P., Spiro, R., Gerold, F., Sessions, R., and Hilaris, B. S. A non-looping afterloading technique for base of tongue implants: results in the first 20 patients. *Int J Radiat Oncol Biol Phys* 11:1853–1855, 1985.

12. Puthawala, A. A., Syed, A. M. N., Neblett, D., and McNamara, C. The role of afterloading iridium implant in the management of the tongue. *Int. J Radiat Oncol Biol Phys* 7:407–412, 1981.

13. Vtyurin, B. M., Ivanov, V. N., Medvedev, V. S., Galantseva, G. F., Abdulkadyrov, S. A., Ivanova, L. F., Petrovskaya, G., and Plichko, V. I. Californium-252 interstitial implants in carcinoma of the tongue. *Int J Radiat Oncol Biol Phys* 11:441–449, 1985.

14. Beiler, D. D. Interstitial radiation in the treatment of carcinoma of the tonsillar region. *Am J Roentgenol Radium Ther Nucl Med* 128:1031–1036, 1977.

15. Mazeron, J. J., Lusinchi, A., Marinello, G., Huart, J., Martin, M., Calitchi, E., Raynal, M., Le Bourgeois, J. P., Baillet, F., and Pierquin, B. Interstitial radiation therapy for squamous cell carcinoma of the tonsillar region: the Creteil experience (1971–1981). *Int J Radiat Oncol Biol Phys* 12:895–900, 1986.

16. Son, Y. H., and Kacinski, B. M. Therapeutic concepts of brachytherapy/megavoltage in sequence for pharyngeal wall cancers. Results of integrated dose therapy. *Cancer* 59: 1268–1273, 1987.

17. Hilaris, B., Lewis, J., and Henschke, U. Therapy of recurrent cancer of the nasopharynx. *Arch Otolaryngol* 87:80–84, 1968.

18. Wang, C. C., Busse, J., and Gitterman, M. A simple afterloading application for intracavitary irradiation of carcinoma of the nasopharynx. *Radiology* 115:737–738, 1975.

19. Vikram, B., and Hilaris, B. Transnasal permanent interstitial implantation of carcinoma of the nasopharynx. *Int J Radiat Oncol Biol Phys* 10:153–155, 1984.

20. Baris, G., Visser, A. G., and van Andel, J. G. The treatment of squamous cell carcinoma of the nasal vestibule with interstitial iridium implantation. *Radiother Oncol* 4:121–125, 1985.

21. Vikram, B., Hilaris, B. S., Anderson, L. L., and Strong, E. W. Permanent iodine-125 implants in head and neck cancer. *Cancer* 51:1310–1314, 1983.

22. Paryani, S. B., Goffinet, D. R., Fee, W. E., Goode, R. L., Levine, P., and Hopp, M. L. Iodine 125 suture implants in the management of advanced tumors in the neck attached to the carotid artery. *J Clin Oncol* 3:809–812, 1985.

23. Martinez, A., Goffinet, D. R., Fee, W., Goode, R., and Cox, R. S. [125]Iodine implants as an adjuvant to surgery and external beam radiotherapy in the management of locally advanced head and neck cancer. *Cancer* 51:973–979, 1983.

CHAPTER 7

Brachytherapy
of
Brain Tumors

Tumors of the brain are a diverse group of lesions that have been historically very difficult to cure by surgery alone. (**Table 7-1.**) Patients with malignant gliomas, which represent the most common primary malignant brain tumor, have been offered greatly increased survival and quality of life by the addition of radiation and chemotherapy to the appropriate surgical resection. Malignant gliomas, despite their locally aggressive behavior, rarely metastasize. Computerized tomography has revolutionized the diagnosis of brain tumors; however, arteriography is still needed in selective cases to determine the blood supply to a tumor before surgery. Histological confirmation is essential since discrepancies in diagnosis can occur when based on preoperative studies; the only exceptions are tumors located in the brain stem and in the deep midline thalamic region. Extensive resection is obviously not possible when the tumor is deep seated or involves the motor or speech area. Irradiation on the order of 5000 to 6000 cGy in 5 to 6 weeks to the whole brain has proven to be of value in prolonging life, although all tumors eventually recur and patients succumb to their disease. Median survival times vary from 28 weeks in patients treated with 5000 cGy to 42 weeks for patients receiving 6000 cGy (BTSG). Delivery of whole brain external radiation in excess of 6000 cGy is frequently accompanied by brain necrosis. Permanent interstitial brachytherapy with doses in excess of 20,000 cGy appears to be significantly less damaging to cerebral vasculature than conventional fractionated external beam radiation in the range of 6000 to 7000 cGy in 6 to 7 weeks.

Interstitial brain brachytherapy has been performed in selected centers for the past 20 years. Brachytherapy is currently recommended for primary or recurrent supratentorial, small to medium size (2 to 6 cm) tumors, with well defined margins.

TABLE 7-1. Brain Tumor Classification

Site of Origin	Incidence (%)
Neuroepithelium	
i.e., Glioblastoma Multiforme	23.0
Astrocytoma	13.0
Ependymoma	2.0
Oligodendrioglioma	1.5
Medulloblastoma	1.5
Miscellaneous	13.0
Nerve sheath	
i.e., Neurolemmoma	6.0
Meninges	
i.e., Meningioma	16.0
Pituitary	8.0
Other (primary)	
i.e., Craniopharyngioma	3.0
Other (metastatic lung, mal. melanoma, breast, kidney, etc.)	13.0

Modified from: *Tumors of the central nervous system*, Geneva; WHO, 1979; Walker, M. Brain and peripheral nerve system tumors. In: *Cancer Medicine*, Holland, J. F., Frei, E. (eds.) Philadelphia: Lea & Febiger, 1973, pp. 1385–1407.

TECHNIQUE

The advent of stereotactic methods, assisted by CT scanning, has made interstitial brachytherapy easier and more accurate. Dose optimization programs to find the best source locations, with computer controlled positioning devices to implement them, have been integrated into these systems.

The Brown-Roberts-Wells (BRW) stereotactic frame illustrated in Chap. 3, is currently employed. The head ring of the stereotactic frame is applied under local anesthesia and is fixed at four points on the patient's skull the day before or, more frequently, on the day the implantation procedure is planned. It permits 3-D localization of points in the CT scan image; and a fairly accurate implementation of the implantation procedure. The patient then undergoes a CT treatment plan scan with contrast enhancement, at 3 to 5 mm intervals throughout the brain (**Fig. 7-1**). This stereotactic method can be used with either a temporary interstitial or a permanent interstitial brachytherapy technique. Ir-192 or I-125 sources are most frequently used for temporary implants; I-125 is almost exclusively used for permanent implants.

Target Volume. The target includes the tumor region, outlined on all CT treatment scan slices, using the outer border of the contrast ring enhancement of the tumor; and a 0.5-cm margin in all directions around the tumor as shown in **Fig. 7-2**. Computerized treatment planning is performed using least square optimization methods to find the best source position, strength, and number of sources required to deliver the planned dose.

Target Dose. A minimum tumor dose of 6000 to 8000 cGy is prescribed at the periphery of the target volume for temporary implants. The source strength and distribution is selected in such a way that a target dose rate of 1000 to 1500 cGy per day is delivered. A target dose of 16,000 to 18,000 cGy is prescribed for permanent I-125 implants.

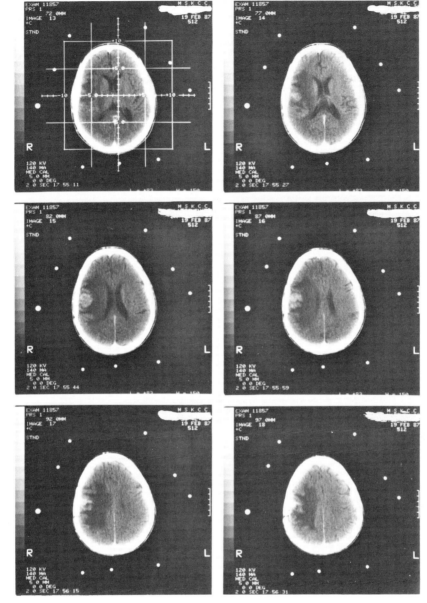

FIGURE 7-1

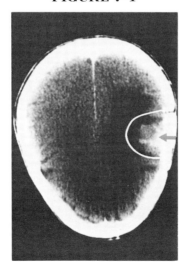

FIGURE 7-2

Temporary Interstitial Implantation Technique

A craniotomy is performed under local anesthesia to allow the insertion of the sources (**Fig. 7-3**, left).

A phantom mount for the stereotactic frame assists in verifying computer generated stereotactic coordinates prior to the actual implantation (Fig. 7-3, right).

These values are set on the stereotactic frame to allow accurate placement of sources within the tumor (**Fig. 7-4**, left). The CT coordinates of target and entry points are translated into stereotactic frame coordinates and approach angles using a computer program (Fig. 7-4, right).

Using the derived stereotactic coordinates, 4 to 8 rigid plastic catheters are inserted into the target volume. The catheters are pushed through the stainless-steel guides of the stereotactic frame. Once in place the catheter is fixed either to the dura or to the skull. The skin incision is closed and the procedure is completed.

On the day following the stereotactic implantation, a CT scan is obtained in as similar a patient position as possible to the pretreatment CT scan to confirm the accurate placement of the sources. Orthogonal localization films are also taken to determine the source relationships. Dose rate contours are then superimposed on both the orthogonal x-rays and the post implantation CT scan.

Patients are isolated in private rooms after Ir-192 implantation. A helmet fashioned from lead foil, which shields the radiation completely, is recommended when I-125 is used. It can be worn by the patient either when visitors or medical personnel enter the room or when the patient wants to walk outside the room.

After the desired dose has been delivered, the patient returns to the operating room and, under local anesthesia, the incision is opened and the sources are removed. The patient is usually discharged on the day following the removal of the sources.

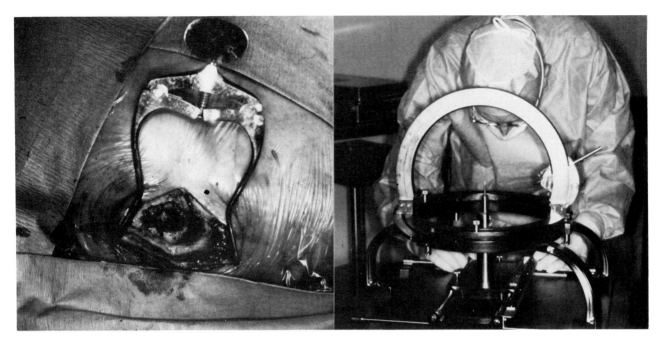

FIGURE 7-3

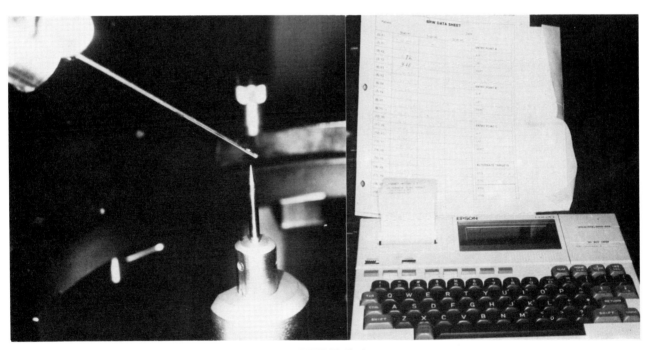

FIGURE 7-4

Permanent Interstitial Brachytherapy Technique

The planning of the procedure is similar to the one described previously for temporary interstitial implants. The New York-Memorial system of dosimetry is used to determine the activity required to deliver 16,000 cGy at the periphery of the target volume. The BRW stereotactic system is employed for the implementation of the implant. Once the stereotactic coordinates are determined and the point of entry is determined on the skull, a modified Mick seed inserter is attached to the stereotactic frame and the required number of seeds are placed in the tumor (**Fig. 7-5**).

Posttreatment CT scan and orthogonal films are taken (see description in temporary implantation technique). Dose contours scaled to match the magnification of the films are produced and superimposed to a CT scan (**Fig. 7-6**, left) and/or orthogonal films (Fig. 7-6, right).

Moorthy et al. have recently (1986) reported the utilization of intraoperative ultrasound guidance of the radioactive sources as an alternative to the stereotactic method. The I-125 seed implantation is carried out using the basic permanent implantation technique (see Chap. 3).

No radiation precautions are necessary for permanent implants. Corticosteroids and anticonvulsant medications are administered when medically indicated.

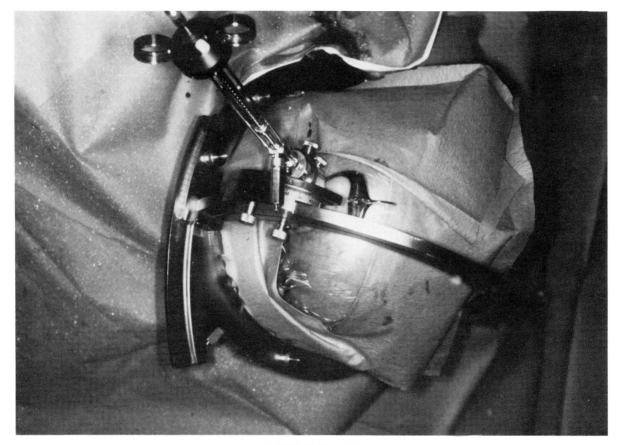

FIGURE 7-5

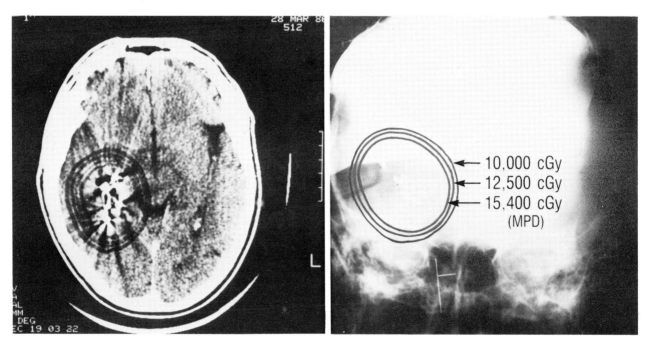

FIGURE 7-6

RESULTS

Stereotactic brain implantation techniques were pioneered in Europe by Talairach, Mundinger, and Szikla. At the University of California, San Francisco, from December 1979 to March 1986, 77 patients with recurrent primary brain tumors underwent I-125 temporary interstitial brachytherapy.

All patients had recurrent malignant gliomas after external radiation and chemotherapy: 42 patients had an anaplastic astrocytoma and 35 had a glioblastoma multiforme (**Table 7-2**). The survival of these patients was superior to a matched group of patients treated with chemotherapy at UCSF.

Although encouraging results have been reported from other European and American centers, it should be emphasized that the interstitial techniques described previously are still being refined. Interstitial brachytherapy has the potential to induce long-term control or even cures; its curative value, however, remains to be proved.

TABLE 7-2.   Experience at the University of California, San Francisco

Tumor Type	Patients at Risk	I-125 Dose (cGY)	Median Survival	2-Year Survial
Anaplastic Astrocytoma	42	5000–12,000	22 months	49%
Glioblastoma Multiforme	35	5000–12,000	17 months	26%

From Phillips et al., 1986.

REFERENCES

1. Kramer, S., Southard, M. E., and Mansfield, C. M. Radiation effect and tolerance of the central nervous system. In: Vaeth, K. (ed.). *Frontiers of Radiation Oncology*, Basel, Switzerland: Karger, 1976, pp. 332–345.

2. Salazar, O. M., Rubin, P., Feldstein, M. L., and Pizzutiello, R. High-dose radiation therapy in the treatment of malignant gliomas: final report. *Int J Radiat Oncol Biol Phys* 5:1733–1740, 1979.

3. Kumar, P. P., Good, R. R., Skultety, M. F., and Carlson, D. T. Absence of deleterious effects of 20,000 to 1,000,000 cGy iodine-125 endocurietherapy on cerebral arteries. *Endocuriether Hyperthermia Oncol* 2:137–146, 1986.

4. Amin, P. P., Salazar, O. M., Salcman, M., Sewchand, W., Drzymala, R., Bellis, E. H., and Wilson, P. D. Stereotactic radioactive brain implants: The opening of a new frontier in neuro-oncology (abstr.). *Int J Radiat Oncol Biol Phys* 11:106 (Supp.), 1985.

5. Chin, H. W., Maruyama, Y., Young, B., Tibbs, P., Markesbery, W., and Goldstein, S. Intracerebral neutron brachytherapy: the technique and application for malignant brain tumors. *Endocuriether Hyperthermia Oncol* 1:222–236, 1985.

6. Frank, F., Gaist, G., Piazza, G., Ricci, R. F., Sturiale, C., and Galassi, E. Stereotactic biopsy and radioactive implantation for interstitial therapy of tumors of the pineal region. *Surg Neurol* 23:275, 280, 1985.

7. Gutin, P. H., Phillips, T. L., Hosobuchi, Y., Wara, M. M., Mackay, A. R., Weaver, K. A., Lamb, S., Hurst, S. Permanent and removable implants for the brachytherapy of brain tumors. *Int J Radiat Oncol Biol Phys* 7:1371–1381, 1981.

8. Gutin, P. H., Phillips, T. L., Wara, W. M., Leikel, S. A., Hosobuchi, Y., Levin, V. A., Weaver, K. A., and Lamb, S. Brachytherapy of recurrent malignant brain tumors with removable high-activity iodine-125 sources. *J Neurosurg* 60:61–68, 1984.

9. Kelly, P. J., Olson, M. H., and Wright, A. E. Stereotactice implantation of iridium 192 into CNS neoplasms. *Surg Neurol* 10:349–354, 1978.

10. Mundinger, F. The treatment of brain tumors with interstitially applied radioactive isotopes. In: Wang, Y., and Pasoletti, P. (eds.). *Radionuclide Applications in Neurology and Neurosurgery*. Springfield, Ill.: Charles C. Thomas, 1970, pp. 199–265.

11. Mundinger, F., and Hoefer, T. Protracted long-term irradiation on inoperable mid-brain tumors by stereotactic curietherapy using iridium-192. *Acta Neurochir [Suppl]* 21:93–100, 1974.

12. Gutin, P. H., and Dormandy, R. H., Jr. A coaxial catheter system for afterloading radioactive sources for the interstitial irradiation of brain tumors. Technical note. *J Neurosurg* 56:734–735, 1982.

13. Findley, P. A., Wright, D. C., Hunington, F. S., Miller, R. W., and Glatstein, E. I-125 interstitial brachytherapy for primary malignant brain tumors: technical aspects of treatment planning and implantation methods (abstr). *Int J Radiat Oncol Biol Phys* 10 (Suppl. 2):98, 1984.

14. Mundiner, F., and Weigel, K. Long-term results of stereotactic interstitial curietherapy. *Acta Neurochir [Suppl]* 33:367–371, 1984.

15. Rao, D. U., Simpson, J. R., Marchosky, J. A., Abrath, F., Henderson, S., and Moran, C. Afterloading interstitial irradiation for CNS tumors (abstr). *Int J Radiat Oncol Biol Phys* 10 (Suppl. 2):144, 1984.

16. Szikla, G., Schlienger, M., Blond, S., Daumas-Duport, C., Missir, O., Miyahara, S., Musolino, A., and Schaub, C. Interstitial and combined interstitial and external irradiation of supratentorial gliomas. Results in 61 cases treated 1973–1981. *Acta Neurochir [Suppl]* 33:355–362, 1984.

17. Schlegel, W., Scharfenberg, H., Doll, J., Pastyr, O., Sturm, V., Netzeband, G., and Lorenz, W. J. CT-images as the basis of operation planning in stereotactical neu-

rosurgery. In: *Proceedings of the First International Symposium on Medical Imaging and Image Interpretation ISMIII 82, Berlin, October 1982*. New York: IEEE, 1982, S. 172–177.

18. Phillips, T. L., Gutin, P. H., and Leibel, S. A. Neurobrachytherapy. State of the art. Henschke Memorial Lecture (abstr.). *Endocuriether Hyperthermia Oncol* 2:207, 1986.

19. Moorthy, C. T., Fakhry, J., Shih, L., and Stern, J. Feasibility of ultrasound-guided iodine-125 brachytherapy for recurrent glioblastoma multiforme (abstr.). *Endocuriether Hyperthermia Oncol* 2:213, 1986.

CHAPTER 8

Brachytherapy in Carcinoma of the Female Breast

Carcinoma of the breast is the most common malignant tumor of women in the Western world. Only 1 percent of breast cancers occur in men. The incidence of breast cancer makes it mandatory to consider any discrete mass, even in young women, as a potential malignancy. Mammography is indicated prior to biopsy because of the possibility of occult cancer in the breast undergoing biopsy, as well as in the other breast. Carcinoma of the breast spreads to regional lymphatics in the axilla, supraclavicular, and infraclavicular regions. Carcinoma of the breast may metastasize to any organ in the body. The most frequently involved sites, however, are the lungs, bones, and liver. Obtaining the level of estrogen receptor protein present in tumor tissue should be considered on all biopsies because this information may be of value in determining subsequent therapy for metastatic disease.

The role of brachytherapy in early breast cancer is as a boost therapy to the area of the primary site, after lumpectomy and external beam radiation. The purpose of treatment is to achieve local control with good cosmetic results. Survival at least equivalent to that obtained with mastectomy is expected. This technique seems to be applicable to the majority of the patients with localized cancer of the breast. The major contraindication to a breast implant is a breast mass located in an area with insufficient surrounding tissue, i.e., in the upper inner quadrant of the breast.

The value of brachytherapy in locally advanced cancer of the breast is limited. Although satisfactory local control may be achieved, severe late radiation effects can be expected, including subcutaneous fibrosis and skin necrosis.

The anatomy of the female breast is shown in **Fig. 8-1**.

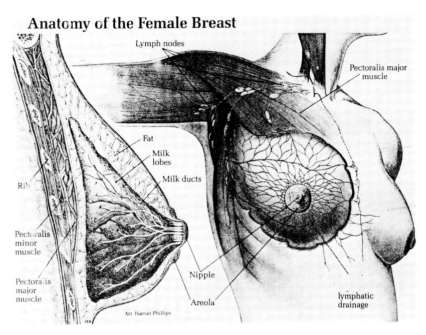

Anatomy of the Female Breast

Lymph nodes

Pectoralis major muscle

Fat

Milk lobes

Milk ducts

Rib

Pectoralis minor muscle

Pectoralis major muscle

Nipple

Areola

lymphatic drainage

Art: Harriet Phillips

FIGURE 8-1

TEMPORARY AFTERLOADING TECHNIQUE

The basic temporary Ir-192 implant technique with a single- or two-plane implant is recommended. The interstitial brachytherapy procedure is performed under general anesthesia with the patient in a supine position and the ipsilateral arm extended over the head.

Prior to the procedure the target volume is drawn on the skin. The number of Ir-192 ribbons required to deliver 1000 to 1500 cGy per day is calculated using the nomograph for a single- or two-plane implant incorporated in the New York–Memorial System of dosimetry. A single-plane implant is adequate if the breast tissue is small; otherwise, a two-plane implant with a separation of 1.5 cm between planes is recommended. To insure a proper implant, the points of insertion of the needles are marked on the skin with a sterile pen (**Fig. 8-2**, left).

Stainless-steel needles are inserted through the skin and spaced parallel at an equal distance, usually 1 to 1.2 cm (Fig. 8-2, right).

The needles are then replaced by plastic tubes (**Fig. 8.3**, left) (see details of the technique in Chap. 3).

Using dummy sources, orthogonal radiographs are taken to define the implanted volume, i.e., the position of the seeds as well as of the markers on the skin for diosimetry. The target volume should be drawn on the radiograph (Fig. 8-3, right).

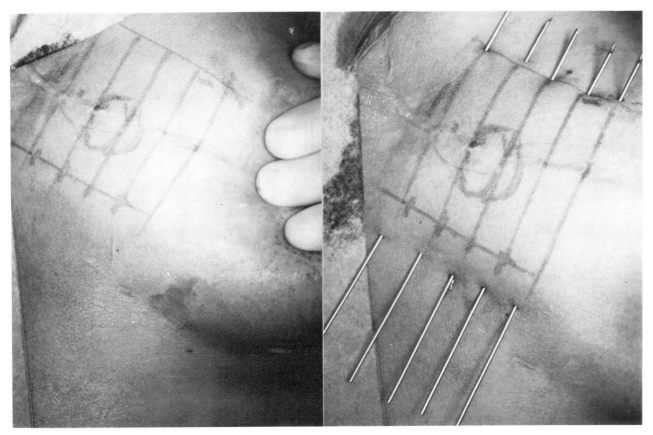

FIGURE 8-2

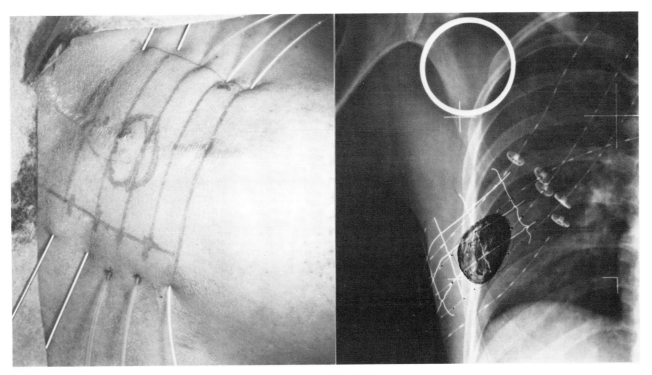

FIGURE 8-3

163

Target Volume.   The target volume, if the procedure is performed after the completion of the external beam radiation, should be estimated on the basis of the size of the primary tumor, the status of the surgical margins, and the type of the closure. An appropriate margin is then outlined and the designated target area is measured and recorded. If the interstitial brachytherapy is to be done immediately after the lumpectomy, however, the tumor volume is marked with surgical clips and an appropriate generous margin is decided (3 to 5 cm) around it.

Target Dose.   If the primary tumor was excised with negative margins a boost target dose of 1200 to 1500 cGy is given. If the margins of resection are involved by tumor, a higher boost dose is delivered in the range of 2000 to 2500 cGy. The typical external course of breast irradiation is 4500 cGy in 25 fractions. The prescription isodose curve must surround all the sources and deliver the planned dose to the target volume (see Chap. 4 for more details).

Two parallel planes of Ir-192 seeds in A/P and lateral projections are shown in **Fig. 8-4**. The isodose distribution perpendicular to the source lines of the implant at various levels (indicated in **Fig. 8-5** A and shown in Fig. 8-5 B–D) are more instructive than distributions in planes parallel either to the lines or to A/P or lateral films.

The loading of the radioactive sources is performed in the patient's room (**Fig. 8-6**). Measurements of the dose with a diode probe or other sensitive radiation detector at multiple points on the skin overlying the implanted region permits isodose-rate contours to be drawn directly on the skin and be compared with computer generated isodose–skin rates (**Fig. 8-7**).

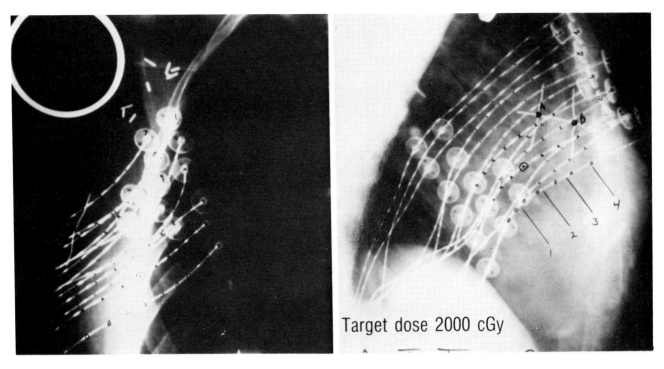

FIGURE 8-4

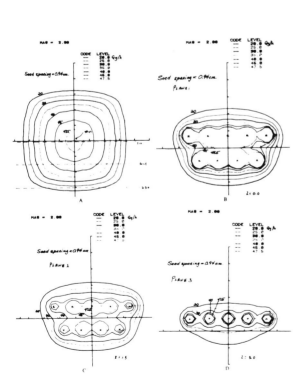

FIGURE 8-5

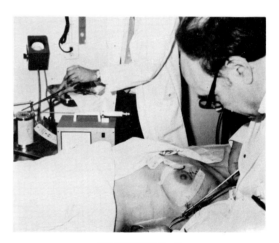

FIGURE 8-6

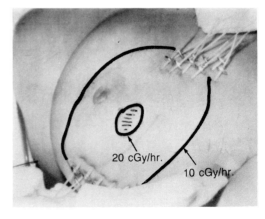

FIGURE 8-7

RESULTS

In 1983 Pierquin et al. reported the Creteil experience in the conservative management of breast cancer. Between 1961 and 1977, 408 patients with T1–T3 tumors were treated; tumors smaller than 3 cm in diameter were excised, while larger tumors were left in place. The local control at 10 years was 92 percent for patients with T1 lesions, 91 percent for T2 lesions, and 85 percent for T3 lesions.

In 1980 Harris et al. reported similarly high 5-year local control rates from the Joint Center for Radiation Therapy using the same technique: 96 percent for stage I and 90 percent for stage II. The implant was done as a separate procedure, after the excision of the primary tumor and external radiation to the whole breast.

In a 1980 retrospective analysis of the RTOG registry patients, Bedwinek et al. found that local control was not a function of tumorectomy if an Ir-192 boost implant was performed (95 percent with tumorectomy and 93 percent without tumorectomy).

In a more recent analysis of the Creteil experience (1986), Leung et al. have shown that identical local control rates could be achieved within each stage with or without tumorectomy (**Table 8-1**), provided that a higher Ir-192 boost dose was given (2500 cGy with tumorectomy; 3700 cGy without tumorectomy).

In 1986, Shank reviewed and compiled long term disease-free survival results for patients with negative nodes, treated with limited surgery and various techniques of radiation, including brachytherapy, showing these results to be equivalent to the results achieved by mastectomy (**Fig. 8-8**).

DISEASE-FREE SURVIVAL IN NODE NEGATIVE (T1 AND T2) PATIENTS TREATED WITH PRESERVATIVE THERAPY

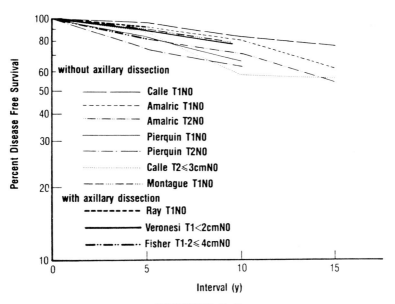

FIGURE 8-8

TABLE 8-1

	Local Control	
	Tumorectomy (%)	No Tumorectomy (%)
Stage		
T1	94.5	96.5
T2	85.0	89.0

REFERENCES

1. Finzi, N. S. Inoperable recurrent carcinoma of the breast under treatment by radium. *Proc R Soc Med* 2:226–227, 1909.

2. Stevenson, W. C. Preliminary clinical report on a new and economical method of radium therapy by means of emanation needles. *Br Med J* 2:9–10, 1914.

3. Janeway, H. H. *Radium Therapy in Cancer at Memorial Hospital, New York.* First report 1915–16. New York: Hoeber, P. B., 1917, pp. 184–190.

4. Keynes, G. The treatment of primary carcinoma of the breast with radium. *Acta Radiol* 10:393–402, 1929.

5. Pfahler, G. E. Results of radiation therapy in 1022 private cases of carcinoma of the breast from 1902 to 1928 (including 127 cases in which radium and roentgen rays were combined). *Am J. Roentgenol* 27:497–508, 1932.

6. Pierquin, B., and Wilson, J. F. Clinical application of iridium-192 in breast cancer. In: *Afterloading: 20 Years of Experience, 1955–1975.* B. S. Hilaris (ed) New York: Memorial Sloan-Kettering Cancer Center, 1975, pp. 113–118.

7. Hilaris, B. S., and Ager, P. J. Cancer of the breast. In: Hilaris, B. S., (ed.). *Handbook of Interstitial Brachytherapy.* Acton, Mass.: Publishing Sciences Group, Inc., 1975, pp. 275–291.

8. Weber, E. T., and Hellman, S. Radiation as primary treatment for local control of breast carcinoma: a progress report. *JAMA* 234:608–611, 1975.

9. Puthawala, A. A., Syed, A. M. N., Sheikh, K. M. A., Gowdy, R. A., and McNamara, C. S. Combined external and interstitial irradiation in the treatment of stage III breast cancer. *Radiology* 153:813–816, 1984.

10. Pierquin, B. Conservative treatment for carcinoma of the breast: experience of Creteil-ten year results. In *Conservative Management of Breast Cancer: New Surgical and Radiotherapeutic Techniques.* In: Harris, J. R., Hellman, S., and Silen, W. (eds.). Philadelphia: JB Lippincott Co., 1983, pp. 11–14.

11. Mansfield, C. M., and Jewell, W. R. Intraoperative interstitial implantation of iridium 192 in the breast. *Radiology* 150:600, 1984.

12. Harris, J. R., Hellman, S., and Kinne D. W. Limited surgery and radiotherapy for early breast cancer. *N Engl J Med* 313:1365–1368, 1985.

13. Shank, B., and Hellman, S. Preservative surgery and radiation therapy in the treatment of early breast cancer. In: Nori, D., and Hilaris, B. S., (eds.), *Radiation Therapy of Gynecological Cancer.* New York: Alan R. Liss, 1987, 251–272.

14. Leung, S., Otmezguine, Y., Calitchi, E. E., Mazeron, J. J., LeBourgeois, J. P., and Pierquin, B. Locoregional recurrences following radical external beam irradiation and interstitial implantation for operable breast cancer—a twenty three year experience. *Radiother Oncol* 5:1–10, 1986.

CHAPTER 9

Brachytherapy for Soft Tissue Sarcomas

BRACHYTHERAPY FOR SOFT TISSUE SARCOMAS

Approximately 5000 new cases of soft tissue sarcomas occur each year in the United States, accounting for less than 1 percent of all neoplasms in adults. They can occur in virtually any of the soft tissues of the body; the most frequent sites, however, are the extremities. Sarcomas are among the most aggressive tumors, spreading extensively along anatomic structures. Conservative resection has been accompanied frequently by local recurrence, and has been abandoned in favor of more radical procedures that, in an extremity, often amount to amputation. External radiation therapy combined with limb preservative surgery has been successful in achieving the same results in small- to medium-size, high-grade tumors as the ones obtained by radical surgical resection. Several studies from Europe and the United States indicate that interstitial brachytherapy combined with function-preserving surgical resection can successfully eradicate microscopic or minimal macroscopic residual sarcomas. This provides alternative solutions for these patients. The theoretical advantages of such a combination include 1) less extensive surgery, 2) synchronous brachytherapy, which allows aggressive treatment of residual malignant cells at a time when these cells are still oxygenated and before they are embedded in healed scar tissue, 3) placing of the implant plane on the residual tumor, which assures this site will receive the highest radiation dose, 4) short treatment (4 to 5 days) completed prior to the discharge of the patient from the hospital, which presents a considerable medical, psychological, and economic

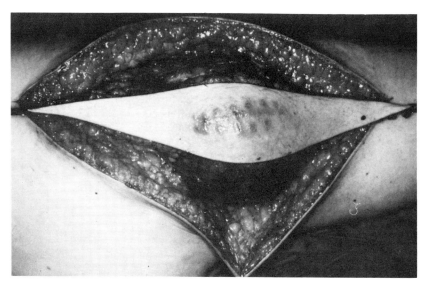

FIGURE 9-1

advantage, and 5) feasibility even when surgery and external beam radiation have previously failed.

Technique.   The basic or the sealed-end temporary implant technique is recommended, depending on the location of the tumor. The surgical treatment consists of an end block resection of the sarcoma and the involved tissue around it, including all previous incisions and biopsy paths (**Fig. 9-1**). The entire specimen is excised in one block without cutting through the tumor if possible. The main aim of resection is not only to remove all tumor, but also to maintain normal function. When the tumor abuts on a major artery, vein, nerve bone, or joint, the structure is carefully dissected off and preserved if technically feasible (**Fig. 9-2**).

Target Volume.   After the surgical removal of the tumor, the overlying skin and soft tissues collapse onto the underlying structures. This composite slab of tissue forms the tumor bed treatment target; it can be flat or uneven. Usually, a single plane implant is found satisfactory. A margin of 2 to 5 cm beyond the boundaries of gross or suspected tumor must be added; the extent of the margin is normally larger along muscles, nerves, and vessels than transverse to those structures. The dimensions of the area to be implanted are measured with a ruler and recorded (**Fig. 9-3**).

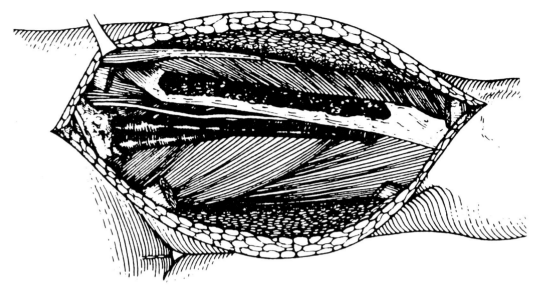

FIGURE 9-2

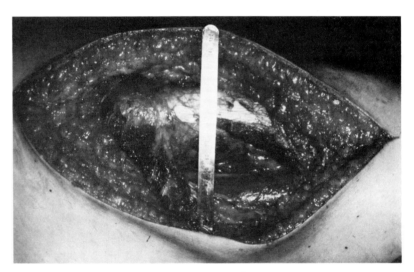

FIGURE 9-3

The number of afterloading tubes that must be placed in the target area in order to deliver 1000 cGy per day is determined using the planar implant nomogram of the New York–Memorial system of dosimetry. The tubes are inserted through normal skin after surgical resection, but before completion of any reconstruction and wound closure. To assure a proper implant, the points of needle insertion are marked on the skin with a sterile pen (**Fig. 9-4**).

Parallel stainless-steel needles are spaced uniformly and embedded in the depth of the operative field. The closed end of each afterloading nylon tube (in the sealed-end technique) is threaded through the needle until it emerges from the opposite end of the needle. The needle is then withdrawn while holding the plastic tube in place until the needle is out of the skin. This process is repeated for the total planned number of afterloading tubes. Each tube is secured in proper position in the tumor bed with #2 or #3 absorbable suture material (**Fig. 9-5**).

Metallic clips are placed near each blind end of the nylon tube for later identification of this end on the localization radiographs. The afterloading tubes are individually secured to the skin by means of a stainless steel button that is threaded over the tube, fixed to it by crimping, and anchored to the underlying skin by silk sutures. A plastic hemispherical bead cushions the button on the skin protecting it from undue pressure.

Wound Closure.   Because of the use of radiation, wound closure requires extra planning and care to avoid undue tension predisposing to wound breakdown (**Fig. 9-6**).

To diminish further the wound complications, the loading of Ir-192 ribbons is delayed until 4 to 5 days after surgery. Prior to loading, anteriorposterior and lateral radiographs with radiopaque markers in the lumens of the plastic tubes provide the information necessary for computerized dosimetry calculations and dose rate determination.

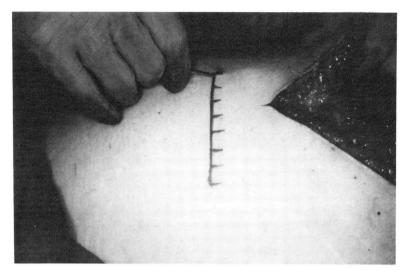

FIGURE 9-4

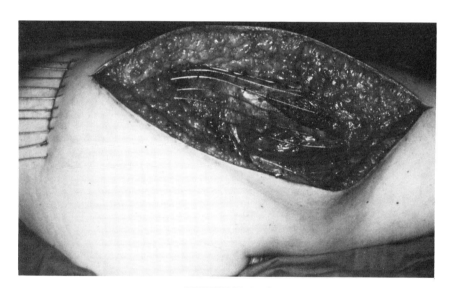

FIGURE 9-5

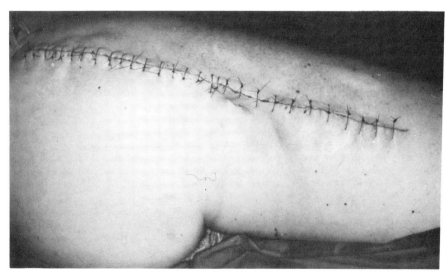

FIGURE 9-6

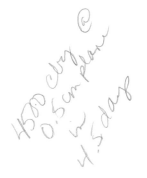

Target Dose. The postimplantation physical evaluation of the implant involves calculating the dose distribution in multiple planes that are roughly perpendicular to the ribbons and selecting the highest dose rate for which the isodose contour is continuous. By dividing the prescribed dose by this treatment dose rate, the treatment time is determined (**Fig. 9-7**, left). The recommended dose for tumor bed implants is 4500 to 5000 cGy/3 to 5 days. The dose distribution around such an Ir-192 implant is shown in a transverse central plane in Fig. 9-7 (right). External radiation should be given if all gross tumor was not resected; in such a case, the implant boost dose is 2500 to 3000 cGy, supplemented by 4000 to 4500 cGy of external beam.

Special Situations. In implants of the leg or in general areas with minimum tissue between the skin and the implant plane, it is important that all drainage tubes are positioned superficially to the nylon tubes, so that they artificially increase the distance between the skin and the radioactive plane. Furthermore these drainage tubes should lie within the field of irradiation so tumor recurrences along their track can be avoided (**Fig. 9-8**, left). Separate determinations of radiation dose are made with a diode probe or other sensitive radiation detector permitting isodose contours to be drawn directly on the skin (Fig. 9-8, right). These measurements are correlated with computer determinations for points of interest, i.e., skin, major vessels, bone, and so on (**Fig. 9-9**). If the projected dose to the normal tissues is more than 4000 cGy over an area of more than 25 cm², or 2500 cGy over an area of more than 100 cm², the target dose should be proportionally decreased until the preceding tolerance doses are met.

1. Obtain the inner continuous curve around plane of implant for each of the standard cuts.

   1._____ Gy/dy
   2._____ Gy/dy
   3._____ Gy/dy   1Gy (gray) = 100 rad
   4._____ Gy/dy
   5._____ Gy/dy

2. Obtain from above the median isodose rate curve. This will be called from now on MPDR (Median Peripheral Dose Rate). _____Gy/d

3. Correlate all isodose curves with the location of the tumor in the x-ray films. Determine whether the tumor is covered properly by the median peripheral dose rate. If yes, proceed to Step #4. If no, go back to Steps 1 to 2 and obtain the next lower curve which will now be called the MPDR._____Gy/d

4. Decide the recommended median peripheral dose (MPD) for the particular patient _____Gy.

5. Divide the MPD in Gy by the MPDR in Gy/d to determine the duration of implantation as _____ days. Multiply this figure by 24 hours to get implantation time = _____ days and _____ hours.

6. Mark on the x-ray film points of interest (e.g. skin, spinal cord, rectum, etc.) for which separate determinations of the radiation dose should be made.

   Points of interest _____   Maximum dose _____Gy
                      _____   _____Gy
                      _____   _____Gy

   _____
   Signature

PATIENT'S NAME: _____   MH#_____

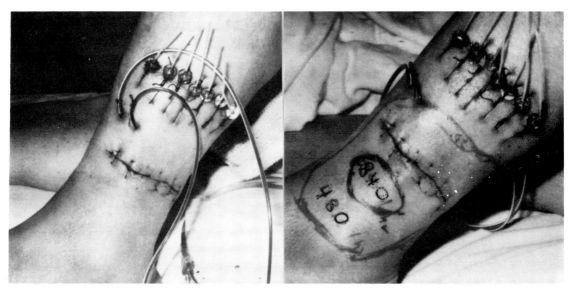

FIGURE 9-7

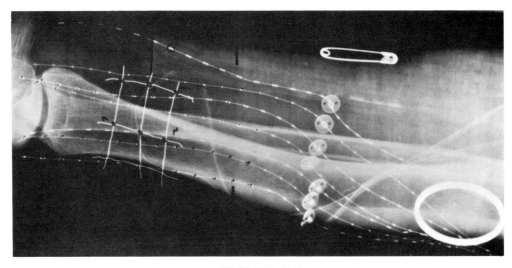

FIGURE 9-8

FIGURE 9-9

Occasionally, in removing a soft tissue sarcoma, a large skin defect is created (**Fig. 9-10**, left upper).

When direct wound closure cannot be achieved without tension in such a large skin defect, a pedicled or myocutaneous flap can be utilized to ensure uncomplicated healing (Fig. 9-10, right upper and left lower).

Such a procedure not only ensures proper wound healing, but maintains a functional arm, as is shown in this example 5 years after brachytherapy and chemotherapy (Fig. 9-10, right lower).

Routine nursing and medical care is provided as usual, but prolonged exposure of staff should be avoided by the sharing of nursing duties and the use of portable lead shields. Upon completion of the planned duration of treatment, the afterloading nylon tubes and the Ir-192 seeds are removed. The puncture sites on the skin require no special care and most of the patients are discharged the following day from the hospital.

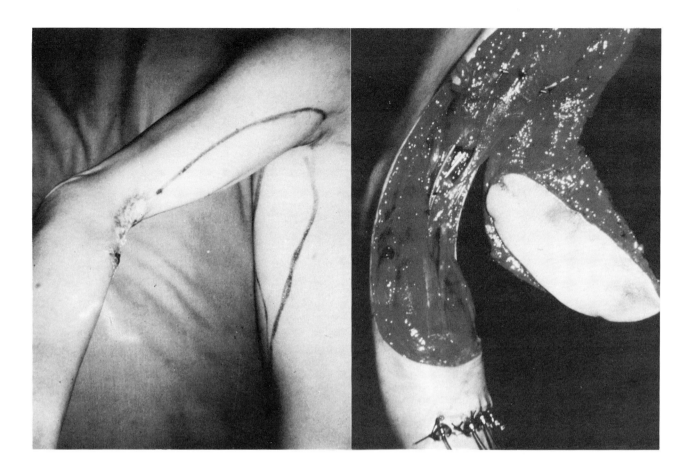

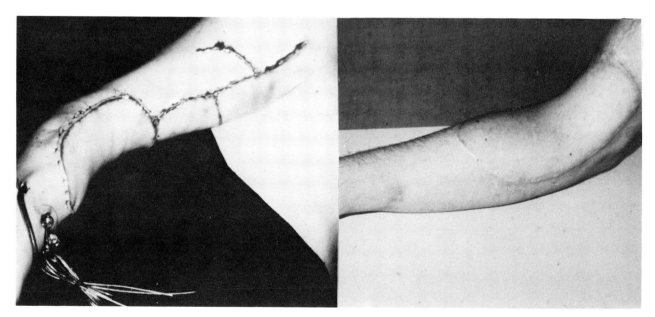

FIGURE 9-10

RESULTS

The early results of this combined limb-sparing resection and brachytherapy approach in patients with locally advanced soft tissue sarcomas of the extremities (**Fig. 9-11**), liposarcomas of the extremities (**Fig. 9-12**), and sarcomas of the popliteal and antecubital fossae (**Fig. 9-13**) demonstrated a low local failure rate comparable to the rates obtained by conservative surgery and external beam therapy. Many of these sarcomas had clinical and pathological features that would have required treatment by amputation. Despite these poor prognostic features, this treatment approach was able to preserve the limb and maintain good function in the majority of the patients.

This treatment technique is currently being evaluated at Memorial Sloan Kettering Cancer Center in a prospective randomized clinical trial together with adjuvant chemotherapy. In an early analysis of complications, it was found that major wound complications were increased in the brachytherapy group compared with the nonbrachytherapy group (22 percent versus 3 percent, $p = 0.002$). No amputations were required, however, and only 14 percent of the brachytherapy-associated wound complications were of prolonged duration (>200 days).

Interim modifications of the brachytherapy procedure, including 1) wound closure utilizing myocutaneous flaps, and 2) extension of the postoperative afterloading interval of Ir-192 sources to a minimum of 5 to 7 days, have contributed to a decrease in the complication rate without sacrificing local control.

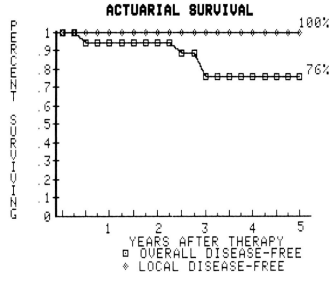

FIGURE 9-11

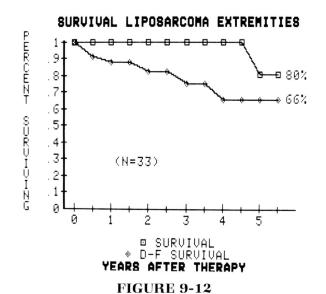

FIGURE 9-12

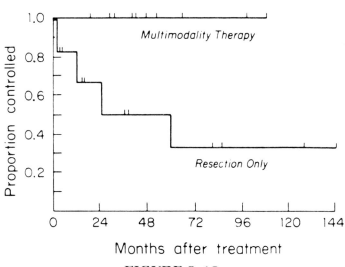

FIGURE 9-13

181

REFERENCES

1. Lindberg, R. D., Martin, R. G., Romsdahl, M. M., and Barkey, H. T. Conservative surgery and postoperative radiotherapy in 300 adults with soft tissue sarcoma. *Cancer* 47:2391–2397, 1981.

2. Suit, H. D., Proppe, K. H., Mankin, H. J., and Wood, W. Preoperative radiation therapy for sarcoma of soft tissue. *Cancer* 47:2269–2274, 1981.

3. Eilber, F. R., Morton, D. L., Eckerdt, J., Grant, T., and Weisenburger, T. Limb salvage for skeletal and soft tissue sarcomas: multidisciplinary preoperative therapy. *Cancer* 53:2579–2584, 1984.

4. Shiu, M. H., Turnbull, A. D., Nori, D., Hajdu, S., and Hilaris, B. S. Control of locally advanced extremity soft tissue sarcomas by function-saving resection and brachytherapy. *Cancer* 53:1385–1392, 1984.

5. Roy, J., Hilaris, B. S., Nori, D., Manolatos, S., Shiu, M. H., Anderson, L. L., Hajdu, S. I., and Brennan, M. F. Adjuvant endocurietherapy in the management of liposarcomas of the extremities. *Endocuriether Hyperthermia Oncol* 2:29–35, 1986.

6. Shiu, M. H., Collin, C., Hilaris, B. S., Nori, D., Manolatos, S., Anderson, L. L., Hajdu, S., Lane, J., Hopfan, S., and Brennan, M. F. Limb preservation and tumor control in the treatment of popliteal and antecubital soft tissue sarcomas. *Cancer* 57:1632–1639, 1986.

7. Brennan, M. F., Shiu, M. H., Collin, C., Hilaris, B. S., Magill, G., Lane, J., Godbold, J., and Hajdu, S. I. Extremity of soft tissue sarcomas. *Cancer Treat Symp* 3:71–81, 1985.

8. Schray, M., Gunderson, L., Sim, F., Pritchard, D., Shives, T., and Yeakel, P. Soft tissue neoplasms: The integration of brachytherapy and external beam irradiation (abstr.). *Endocuriether Hyperthermia Oncol* 2:214, 1987.

9. Arbeit, J. M., Hilaris, B. S., and Brennan, M. F. Wound complications in the multimodality treatment of extremity and superficial truncal sarcomas. *J Clin Oncol* 5 (3):480–488, 1987.

10. Brennan, M. F., Shiu, M. H., Collin, C., Hilaris, B., Magill, G., Lane, J., Godbold, J., and Hajdu, S. I. Extremity soft tissue sarcomas. *Cancer Treat Symp* 3:71–82, 1985.

CHAPTER 10

Clinical Applications in Cancer of the Lung

In this century, the United States is experiencing what can be best described as an epidemic of lung cancer. The incidence and mortality rates have risen steadily every year. Survival rates during the same period have improved, but even by the best estimates only one out of eight lung cancer patients is expected to survive for 5 years.

Carcinoma of the lung includes squamous cell carcinoma, adenocarcinoma, large cell carcinoma, and small cell carcinoma. Adenocarcinoma is on the increase so that it may be the most common histological type. All four histological types can metastasize, although at seemingly different rates and to different locations, even before the tumor has reached a detectable size, i.e., to the regional (hilar and mediastinal) lymph nodes, as well as to distant sites, such as the brain, bone, adrenals, and liver. A lymph node map is used in our Center to help identify the different levels of mediastinal lymph nodes (**Fig. 10-1**).

The treatment of choice for operable nonsmall cell lung cancer is surgical resection. A small percentage of patients with nonsmall-cell cancer is suitable for intensive radiation therapy. Local thoracic external beam irradiation, however, is limited by the tolerance of vital organs that lie within the treatment area. Interstitial brachytherapy helps the radiation oncologist to overcome the limitations imposed by the normal tissues. At the same time, the closer the relationship between the radiation and the surgical oncologist allows for a better intraoperative tumor assessment and a more effective combined therapy.

Interstitial brachytherapy has a good curative potential in patients with localized small- to moderate-sized nonsmall-cell lung tumors that are well defined, have not metastasized to lymph nodes, and are easily accessible so that they can be adequately implanted. Larger tumors, multiple lesions, or the presence of lymph node metastases preclude curative treatment by implantation. In selected cases, quick and effective palliation may be obtained by an intraoperative, percutaneous, or endobronchial interstitial implant.

Table 10-1 lists the various brachytherapy approaches in the treatment of nonsmall-cell lung cancer. The brachytherapy technique used depends

SITES OF LYMPH NODES

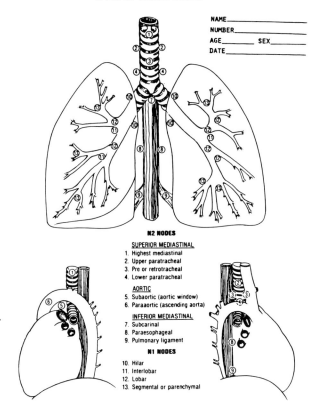

FIGURE 10-1

TABLE 10-1

Approach	*Clinical Application*
Intraoperative Permanent I-125	discrete lung or mediastinal masses
Intraoperative Temporary Ir-192	chest wall or very small mediastinal lesions
Permanent I-125 Vicryl suture	discrete chest wall or mediastinal lesions or postive margins of resection
transbronchial I-125	small tracheal or main bronchus lesions
Intraluminal remote afterloading	minimal tracheal or bronchial disease; positive margins of resection

on the tumor location and the amount of gross disease. Discrete lung masses or mediastinal lymph nodes are permanently implanted with I-125 seeds. Chest wall and small mediastinal lesions or positive margins of resection are treated by either temporary Ir-192 implants or I-125 absorbable Vicryl suture seeds. Endobronchial tumors are managed transbronchially by either a permanent I-125 implant or by an intraluminal, preferably remotely controlled, application.

INTRAOPERATIVE PERMANENT INTERSTITIAL TECHNIQUE

Patients selected for this procedure must have adequate pulmonary function so that they can tolerate thoracotomy without major risk. They should also have nonsmall cell tumors localized to the hemithorax without pleural invasion or effusion and without evidence of distant metastases.

The majority of the permanent interstitial implants of the lung are performed through a posteriolateral approach, which is the usual approach when resection of a lung cancer is contemplated. This approach has been found to be very satisfactory because it permits a good exposure of the tumor to be implanted and allows inspection of the hilar area and the ipsilateral mediastinum. It is unsatisfactory, however, for tumors extending to the contralateral hilum or mediastinum. A small anterior thoractomy incision may be used in this instance, but the exposure is generally not adequate for an effective implantation of all tumors. The thoracic surgeon must provide an adequate exposure and determine that the lung tumor is not resectable, at which point the radiation oncologist joins the operating team and decides on the basis of the tumor extent and other factors if an interstitial implant is indicated (**Table 10-2**).

Basic Permanent Implantation Technique

The first step of this afterloading technique consists of the insertion of stainless-steel needles into the tumor (**Fig. 10-2**, left); the second step is the afterloading of the needles with the radioactive sources (Fig. 10-2, right). Refer to Chap. 3 for more information on this technique.

The method of determining the target volume dimensions has been described in Chap. 4. The suggested steps for determining the number of I-125 seeds, the spacing of the seeds along each needle (preferably 0.5 cm), and the spacing between needles using the nomograph for permanent I-125 implantation is also described in Chap. 4, to which the reader should refer for more details.

The number of needles required is determined by dividing the number of seeds to be used by the number of seeds planned for each needle. Having determined the number of needles required for the procedure, the brachytherapist's hand is introduced posterior to tumor mass. The required number of needles is then inserted into the tumor, using the selected spacing, until each needle tip can be felt by the examining finger, at which point the needle is pulled back for approximately 0.5 cm—a distance equal to the length of a seed.

TABLE 10-2

Factors	Indications for Intraoperative Basic Permanent Interstitial Brachytherapy
Age	Any
Pulmonary function	FEV1: < 1.2 Liter
Histology	Nonsmall Cell cancer
Grade	Well to moderate differentiated
Tumor size	Less than 6 cm
Localized direct invasion to mediastinum	Acceptable
Nodes	Hilar or resectable mediastinal
Pleural effusion	Not present
Distant metastases	Not present

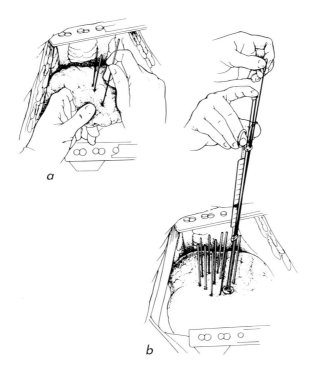

FIGURE 10-2

The applicator is now attached to a peripheral needle with the aid of an Adson clamp, and I-125 seeds are inserted through the needle according to the selected spacing. After the insertion of the precalculated number of seeds, the needle is removed and detached from the inserter. The process is repeated with each needle until all the needles have been loaded (**Fig. 10-3**, left—schematic drawing; right—actual procedure).

During the implantation, a careful record of the number of implanted I-125 seeds, the activity per seed, and the spacing between seeds along each needle should be kept.

On the average, the procedure adds 45 minutes to 1 hour to the operating time. It does not increase hospital stay, it does not increase significantly postoperative morbidity, and it converts an exploratory thoracotomy into an immediate therapeutic procedure.

Target Volume. Includes the palpable and/or radiographically demonstrated tumor and a minimum of 1 cm margin around it. Enlarged hilar nodes are included in the target volume; however, if they cannot be implanted by this technique, the remaining radioactivity is implanted using the Vicryl suture technique (see below).

Target Dose. This is calculated by the New York–Memorial System of dosimetry. It ranges from 16000 cGy for tumors larger than 3 cm to 32000 cGy for tumors about 1.5 to 2.0 cm.

Permanent Vicryl Suture or Gelfoam-Impregnated I-125 Seeds Technique

Both techniques are useful in chest wall lesions, small residual tumors in the mediastinum, or suspicious margins after resection (Chap. 3). A curved needle attached to the Vicryl suture facilitates the anchoring of the suture on the tissues. When the residual tumor is inadequate or near vulnerable structures a Gelfoam plaque or Vicryl/Dexon mesh, available in most of the operating rooms, can be used. The latter technique is illustrated in **Fig. 10-4**; suturing of the Vicryl suture on the Vicryl/Dexon mesh (left) and subsequent attachment to the superior mediastinum (right).

Target Volume. This includes the visible or suspected tumor and a minimum of 1 cm around it.

Target Dose. This is 16000 cGy calculated by the New York–Memorial System of dosimetry.

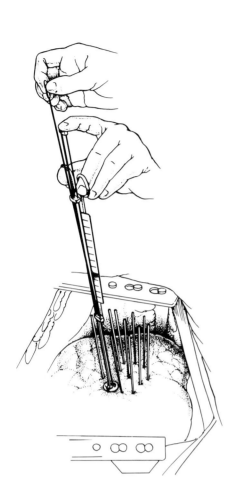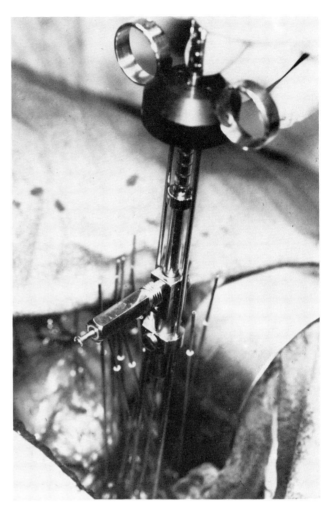

FIGURE 10-3

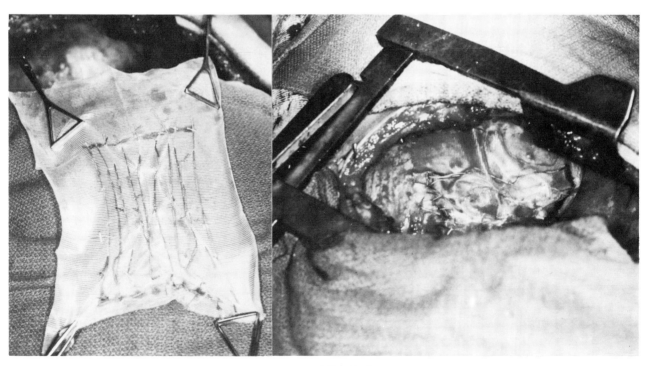

FIGURE 10-4

Results in Early Nonsmall-Cell Lung Cancer Only a limited number of reports in the literature refer to the results of radiation therapy with curative intent in early lung cancer. Although the number of patients reported in each of these series is small, the results suggest that radiation therapy aimed at cure may be a satisfactory alternative to surgery for patients with small lesions and negative mediastinal nodes who cannot tolerate resection.

From 1958 to 1984, inclusive, 55 patients with nonsmall-cell lung cancer with negative nodes (41 pts) or hilar only nodes (14 pts) underwent interstitial brachytherapy at Memorial Sloan-Kettering Cancer Center, instead of resection, mainly because of irreversible obstructive pulmonary disease. All small lesions (T1N0) were localled controlled; 70 percent of the larger lesions or lesions involving hilar nodes (T2N0 or T1-2N1) (**Fig. 10-5** left). The overall actuarial 5-year survival was 32 percent; the 5-year local disease-free survival was 63 percent. There was no statistically significant difference in survival between patients with tumors less than 3 cm (T1) and more than 3 cm (T2) (Fig. 10-5, right).

An example of permanent interstitial brachytherapy in a patient with epidermoid carcinoma in the right upper lobe and negative nodes (T1N0) is shown in **Fig. 10-6**; 2 months after treatment (left) and 11 years after treatment (right). This patient died 2 years later of myocardial infarction without evidence of cancer.

Another example of permanent insterstitial brachytherapy in a patient with adenocarcinoma in the left upper lobe and hilar nodal disease (T2N1M0) is shown in **Fig. 10-7**; before treatment (left) and 64 months after treatment (right). This patient is alive and free of disease as of the time of this report.

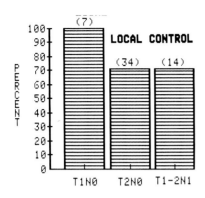
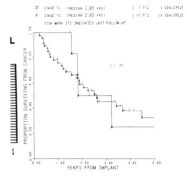

FIGURE 10-5

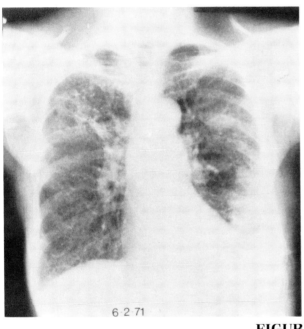
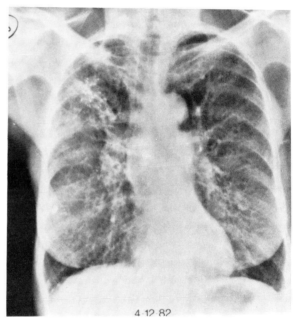

6·2·71   4·12·82

FIGURE 10-6

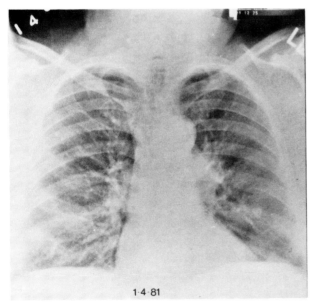
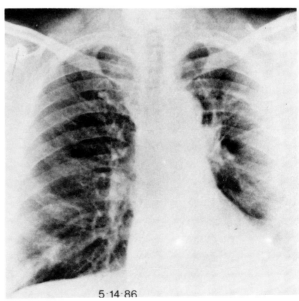

1·4·81   5·14·86

FIGURE 10-7

Results in Advanced Localized Nonsmall-Cell-Lung Cancer. Between 1977 and 1980, 88 patients with involved mediastinal nodes were treated by a permanent I-125 interstitial implant of the primary lung lesion and a temporary Ir-192 implant of the superior mediastinum. Most of these patients (66/88) received postoperative external radiation to the mediastinum and/or the primary site; the midplane dose ranged from 3000 cGy in 2 weeks to 4000 cGy in 4 weeks. The median survival was 26 months and the 2-year survival 51 percent. Locoregional control was observed in 76 percent of the patients (67/88).

The effects of interstitial brachytherapy are limited to the irradiated volume and, therefore, the damage to the surrounding normal lung tissue is less than when external radiation is used. This was shown to be true in all patients who have survived more than 2 years and in whom the lung cancer was locally controlled. A typical example is shown in **Fig. 10-8**; a chest x-ray demonstrating a large right upper lobe lesion with involvement of the mediastinum (left), and the same patient 3 years after an I-125 implant of the primary tumor (16,000 cGy) and postoperative mediastinal radiation (4000 cGy/4 weeks). The patient is alive without evidence of disease as of the time of this report.

Results in Superior Sulcus Tumors. From 1960 to 1982, 129 patients with superior sulcus tumor underwent a thoracatomy at Memorial Sloan-Kettering Cancer Center. A detailed analysis of this group of patients was recently published. Of the 129 patients, 103 had residual or unresectable tumors at thoracotomy and were treated with either a permanent I-125 implant or an Ir-192 temporary implant. Pre- or postoperative external beam radiation was given to the majority of these patients (2000 cGy/1 week or 4000 cGy/4 weeks). Approximately 70 percent of the treated patients were locally controlled. The median survival was 19 months.

The relatively good local control can be explained on the basis of the high target dose that is delivered with a permanent I-125 implant (**Fig. 10-9**, left). At the same time the marked decrease of the radiation dose outside the implanted volume (in this example a tenfold decrease within 2 cm) contributes to the fairly well localized late fibrosis, which is asymptomatic in the majority of the patients, and to the lack of severe brachial neuritis (Fig. 10-9, right).

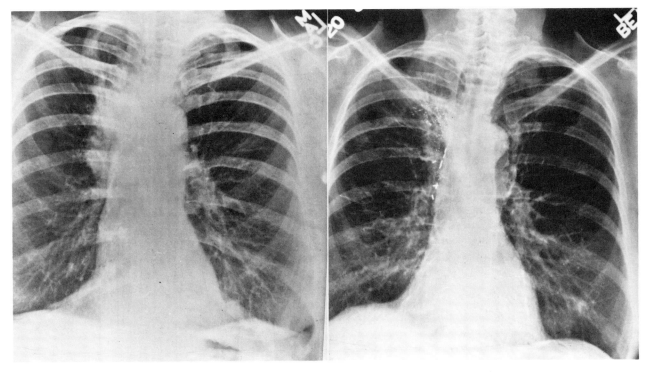

FIGURE 10-8

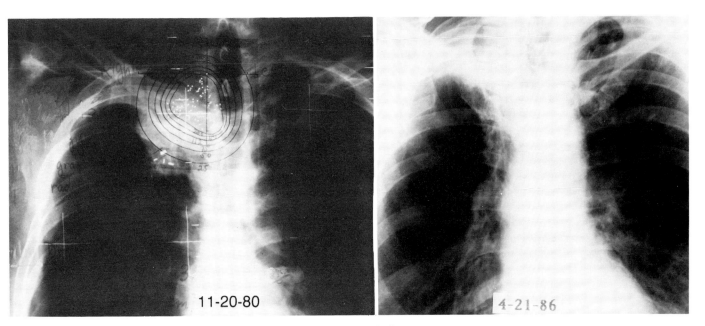

FIGURE 10-9

193

INTRAOPERATIVE TEMPORARY INTERSTITIAL TECHNIQUE

Patients are selected for this procedure either because they have positive superior mediastinal nodes following a complete resection of the primary tumor, but an incomplete mediastinal dissection, and are felt to be poor candidates for locoregional control by postoperative external radiation therapy alone, or because they have chest wall tumors with minimal residual disease or microscopically positive margins after resection.

Technique

The sealed-end technique is utilized (Chap. 3). The tumor is inspected and the width and length of the area to be implanted are measured with a caliper. The number of afterloading plastic catheters required to be placed in the target area is determined by using the planar Ir-192 implant guide of the New York–Memorial system of dosimetry (Chap. 4). The hilar vessels and the major structures of the mediastinum, including the trachea, esophagus, vena cava, aorta, and phrenic and vagal nerves, are identified and their positions are clearly noted in order to avoid injury to these structures at the time of placement of the afterloading plastic tubes. The skin on the anterior chest wall, between the nipple and the anterior axillary line, is marked with a sterile pen to indicate the points through which the catheters will be passed into the chest. A hollow, preferably curved or straight stainless-steel needle (Chap. 2) is inserted into the chest through the planned mark on the skin. The closed end of the plastic tube is threaded through the needle until it emerges from the opposite end of the needle. The needle is then removed while holding the plastic tube in the chest and pulling the needle out through the chest wall. In this manner the process is repeated for the planned number of afterloading tubes. Each tube is placed in the desired position in the mediastinum or chest wall and secured with a #2 or #3 chromic or Dexon absorbable suture material (**Fig. 10-10**, left). The afterloading tubes are fixed to the skin by threading a plastic hemisphere through the projecting end of the tube, followed by a stainless-steel button. The stainless-steel button is then secured to the skin with silk suture (Fig. 10-10, right). Metallic clips are placed near the closed end of each tube within the chest for later identification of this end on the localization radiographs (**Fig. 10-11**, left).

Target Volume.   Includes the tumor area and a 1-cm margin at least around it. In mediastinal implants the target volume includes the entire superior mediastinum.

Target Dose.   A minimal dose of 3000 cGy is prescribed (Fig. 10-11, right) and is supplemented by 4500 to 5000 cGy external beam radiation. The evaluation of the dosimetric calculations and the determination of the implantation time is done according to the guidelines described in Chap. 4. This combined treatment is well tolerated as is demonstrated in **Fig. 10-12**, an x-ray of the same patient taken 5 years after the combined treatment.

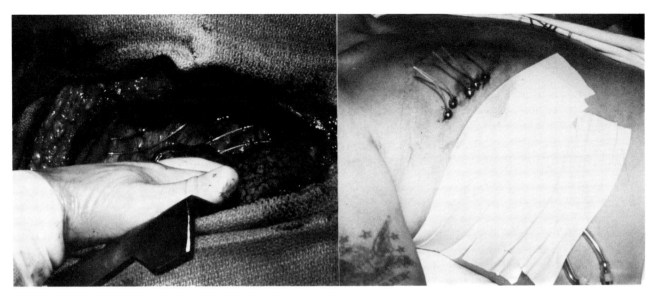

FIGURE 10-10

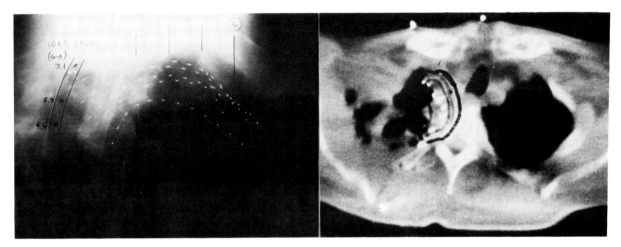

FIGURE 10-11

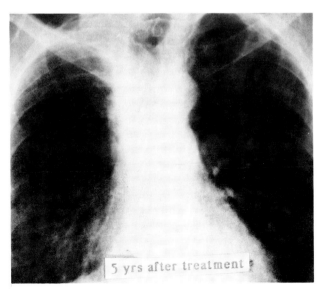

FIGURE 10-12

PERCUTANEOUS PERMANENT INTERSTITIAL TECHNIQUE

There are a number of patients who would ordinarily be candidates for permanent interstitial brachytherapy, but who cannot tolerate a thoracotomy or are reluctant to undergo such a procedure. It is in this group that percutaneous implantation using CT scans and fluoroscopic guidance is recommended. This technique is applicable to patients with tumors abutting or attached to pleura and chest wall in order to minimize the incidence of pneumothorax and intrapulmonary hemorrhage.

Technique

The basic permanent I-125 interstitial technique is used. CT scans are obtained within 4 to 5 days before the procedure and include 3- or 5-mm thick contiguous cuts through the entire tumor with sagittal and coronal reconstruction. These images allow precise delineation of tumor location and volume. In addition, they enable the medical physicist to develop a treatment plan that includes the number of required seeds, their location within the tumor, and radioactivity necessary to achieve the planned target dose; the number of needles, and depth of placement of each needle; and finally, the number of seeds to be placed through each needle.

The procedure is performed in the biplane fluoroscopy room with the patient in the appropriate position necessary to approach the tumor (**Fig. 10-13**, left). the skin surface and the subcutaneous and deep chest wall tissues to the level of the tumor are infiltrated by a local anesthetic. Standard stainless-steel brachytherapy needles are then inserted into the tumor according to the treatment plan (Fig. 10-13, right). To avoid puncture of the intercostal vessels the needles should be introduced along the superior surface of the ribs. The position of each needle is checked by fluoroscopy to make sure that complies with the treatment plan, and if necessary is corrected. The loading of the needles with the radioactive seeds is accomplished with the special inserter; and the needles are removed (**Fig. 10-14**, left). Orthogonal radiographs are usually taken at the completion of the procedure for the final dosimetric studies (Fig. 10-14, right).

This technique provides effective treatment of local disease, as is demonstrated in **Fig. 10-15.** The photograph on the left is taken prior to treatment; the photograph on the right is taken 6 months after treatment, and it shows a marked tumor resolution. This technique does not require general anesthesia, there is no requirement for overnight hospital admission, morbidity has been minimal, and it is cost effective.

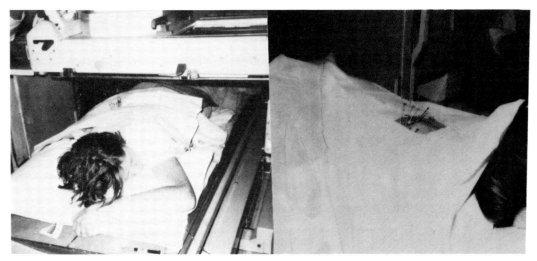

FIGURE 10-13

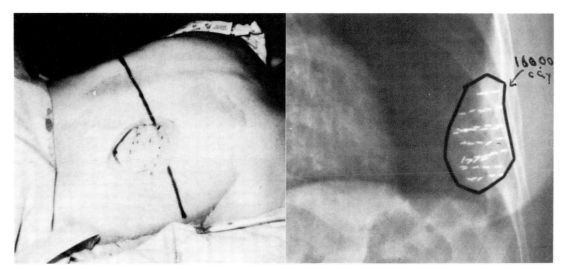

FIGURE 10-14

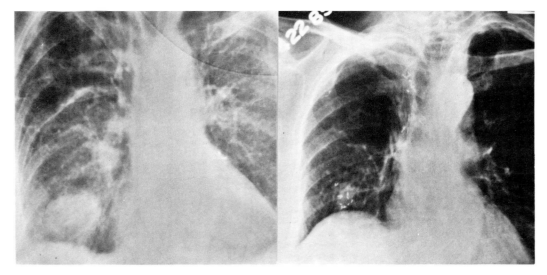

FIGURE 10-15

ENDOTRACHEAL/ENDOBRONCHIAL INTRACAVITARY TECHNIQUE

There is little that can be offered to patients who present with recurrence in the trachea or major bronchi following extensive surgery and/or external beam radiation. Most of these patients have hemoptysis and airway obstruction, often severe enough to cause near asphyxia. To open the airway or to control hemorrhage, transbronchial resection, cauterization, cryosurgery, endobronchial brachytherapy, and, more recently, photoirradiation with laser beams have been used.

Technique

The technique utilizes high dose rate remote afterloading and is performed under sedation and local anesthesia, usually on an outpatient basis (**Fig. 10-16**, left). Thirty milliliters of viscous xylocaine or a similar local anesthetic is given to the patient to swallow and an additional amount in form of a spray is used every 15 minutes when needed. The trachea is anesthetized by injecting 4 percent lidocaine through the cricothyroid membrane.

A flexible bronchoscope with an endotracheal tube attached to its proximal end is advanced alongside and beyond the endotracheal or endobroncheal lesion for inspecting the tumor at all levels, and is then held just beyond the most distal margin of the tumor (Fig. 10-16, right).

The endotracheal tube is advanced over the fiberoptic bronchoscope until its distal end is proximal to the tumor. The endotracheal tube is taped to the skin. The point at the bronchoscope exit from the endotracheal tube is marked. The flexible bronchoscope is removed, and the length from the mark to the tip of the bronchoscope is measured. The same distance as on the flexible bronchoscope is marked on the afterloading catheter used for the treatment (**Fig. 10-17**, left).

A smaller diameter catheter with lead marks, spaced 1 cm from center to center, is introduced into the afterloading catheter to be used for localization and dosimetry purposes. The afterloading catheter is now introduced into the endotracheal tube and pushed down until the mark reaches the beginning of the endotracheal tube (Fig. 10-17, right).

Localization radiographs (A P and lateral) are taken, the target region is outlined with the help of the lead marker images, and the dose prescription is completed (**Fig. 10-18**, left). The afterloading catheter is then connected to the remote afterloading machine, and the treatment begins (Fig. 10-18, right).

Target Volume. The length of the segment to be irradiated is determined by using the radiograph. A margin of at least 2 cm should be added to the proximal and distal margins of the tumor.

Target Dose. A dose of 500 cGy at 1 cm from the linear source is prescribed and repeated weekly for 5 to 6 fractions.

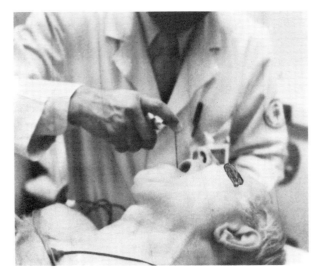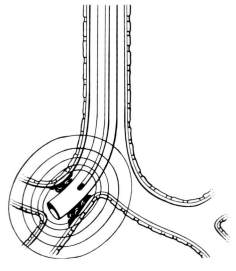

FIGURE 10-16

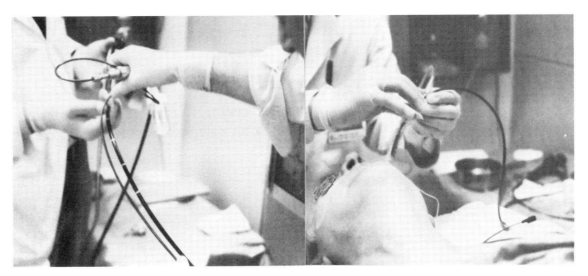

FIGURE 10-17

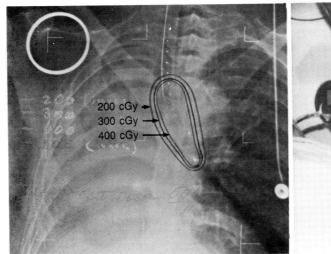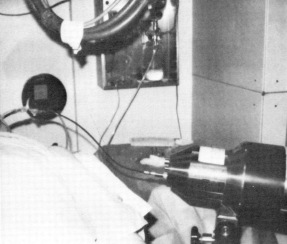

200 cGy
300 cGy
400 cGy

FIGURE 10-18

Esophageal Intracavitary Technique

A remote afterloading technique, similar to the technique described previously for endobronchial applications, is used for the treatment of cancer of the esophagus.

Procedure. The planning of the treatment is based on CT scan, esophagogram, and endoscopic visualization of the tumor location and extent. More recently, the availability of endoscopic ultrasound allows a more accurate determination of the tumor depth. The procedure is performed on an outpatient basis under local anesthesia or sedation. The patient is then placed on his or her side to facilitate the introduction of the special afterloading tube used for treatment. This tube is 4 mm in diameter and incorporates a radiopaque marker at its distal end (**Fig. 10-19**, left).

To make the introduction of the afterloading catheter into the esophagus easier, a short piece, 4 to 5 cm in length, is cut from the distal end of a #16-gauge Foley catheter and is attached to the distal end of the afterloading tube (Fig. 10-19, right).

The afterloading tube is slowly advanced into the esophagus, while the patient is asked to swallow; it is pushed 3 to 4 cm beyond the distal margin of the lesion. The proximal end of the catheter is then connected to the treatment unit (**Fig. 10-20**, left). The treatment parameters (active length of treatment, dose per fraction, and depth of dose prescription) are entered into the computer, and the treatment begins.

Target Volume. Includes the tumor and 3 to 4 cm above and below it.

Target Dose. The target dose is 1500 to 2000 cGy at 1 cm depth, in 3 to 4 applications spaced once-a-week apart, is given for palliation. If the intracavitary treatment is combined with external beam therapy, 2 fractions of 700 cGy each are given at a distance of 1 cm from the source 2 to 3 weeks after a dose of 5000 cGy external beam.

Figure 10-20 (middle) is an example of a 5-cm esophageal lesion recurrent after external radiation; the photograph next to it (Fig. 10-20, right) shows an esophagogram of the same patient 6 months after 1500 cGy remote afterloading intracavitary irradiation, with no evidence of disease.

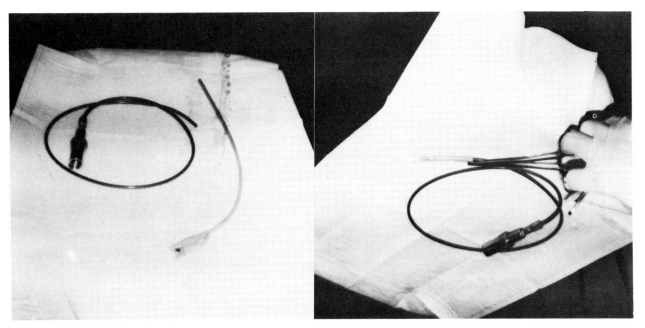

FIGURE 10-19

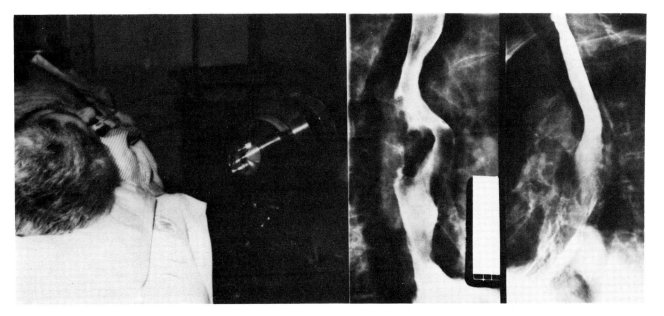

FIGURE 10-20

REFERENCES

1. Graham, E. A., and Singer, J. J. Successful removal of an entire lung for carcinoma of the bronchus. *JAMA* 101:1371–1374, 1933.

2. Henschke, U. K. Interstitial implantation in the treatment of primary bronchogenic carcinoma. *Am J Roentgenol Radium Ther Nucl Med* 79:981–987, 1959.

3. Hilaris, B. S., and Martini, N. Interstitial brachytherapy in cancer of the lung: a 20-year experience. *Int J Radiat Oncol Biol Phys* 5:51–56, 1979.

4. Hilaris, B. S., and Martini, N. Multimodality therapy of superior sulcus tumors. In: Bonica, J. J., Ventafridda, V., Pagni, C. A., Jones, L. E. (eds.). *Advances in Pain Research and Therapy*. New York: Raven Press, 1982, 4:113–122.

5. Hilaris, B. S., Nori, D., Hopfan, S., Batata, M., Bains, M. S., and Martini, N. Endobronchial brachytherapy. In: Hilaris, B. S. and Nori, D. (eds.). *Brachytherapy Oncology—1982*. New York: Memorial Sloan-Kettering Cancer Center, 1982, pp. 47–52.

6. Hilaris, B. S., Nori, D., Beattie, E. J., Jr. and Martini, N. The value of perioperative brachytherapy in the management of non-oat cell carcinoma of the lung. *Int J Radiat Oncol Biol Phys* 9:1161–1166, 1983.

7. Nag, S. Brachytherapy for lung cancer: review. *Cancer Treat Symp* 2:49–56, 1985.

8. Hilaris, B. S., and Nori, D. Intraoperative therapy for non-resectable disease. In: Delarue, N. C., and Eschapasse, H. (eds.). *International Trends in General Thoracic Surgery* 1 (19):207–216, 1985, WB Saunders, Philadelphia.

9. Horowitz, B. S., Young, D. O., Bae, C., Lewis, J. W., and Winchester, M. B. Interstitial irradiation of non-oat cell carcinoma (abstr.). *Endocuriether Hyperthermia Oncol* 2:63, 1986.

10. Hilaris, B. S., Nori, D., and Martini, N. Results of radiation therapy in stage I and II unresectable non small cell lung cancer. *Endocuriether Hyperthermia Oncol* 2 (1):15–21, 1986.

11. Hilaris, S. New approaches in radiation therapy of lung cancer. *Chest* 89(4):349S, 1986.

12. Hilaris, B. S., Nori, D., and Martini, N. Intraoperative radiotherapy in stage I and II lung cancer. *Semin Surg Oncol* 3:22–32, 1987.

13. Hilaris, B. S., and Nori, D. Status of radiotherapy in the management of nonsmall cell lung cancer. *Oncology* 1(2):25–31, 1987.

14. Heelan, R. T., Hilaris, B., Anderson, L., Nori, D., Martin, N., Watson, R. C., Caravelli, J. F., and Linares, L. Percutaneous I-125 seed implantation of lung tumors using computed tomography: early experience. *Radiology* 164: 735–740, 1987.

15. Hilaris, B. S., Martini, N., Wong, G. Y., and Nori, D. Treatment of superior sulcus tumor (Pancoast tumor). In: *Surgical Clinics of North America*. Philadelphia: WB Saunders, Vol. 67, (5), 965–977, 1987.

CHAPTER 11

Brachytherapy
for
Cancer of the Pancreas

Cancer of the pancreas is a common and lethal malignancy. The incidence of this cancer continues to rise and now ranks as the fourth leading cause of cancer death in the United States. In the absence of jaundice, symptoms are vague and nonspecific. In general, tumors of the periampullary region and the adjacent head of the pancreas cause epigastric pain and jaundice; while cancer of the body causes back pain. Imaging techniques such as CT scan and abdominal ultrasound help to diagnose accurately pancreatic malignancy preoperatively. Surgery remains the primary approach to exocrine carcinoma, but resectability rates are low with few long-term survivors. Carcinoma of the pancreas is often unresectable because of invasion of the adjacent major blood vessels. The need for meaningful palliation remains a challenge. The use of conventional external beam radiation in the primary treatment of pancreatic carcinoma has been of minimal benefit in prolonging survival or achieving palliation of pain. Intraoperative interstitial brachytherapy into localized unresectable pancreatic tumors has been suggesgted as a means of achieving palliation of pain and local control without significant complications or operative mortality.

Technique

The basic permanent interstitial technique is used. Under general anesthesia an exploratory laparatomy is performed. The laparatomy allows an accurate determination of the extent of disease within the pancreas and into adjacent peripancreatic tissues or to other areas in the abdomen

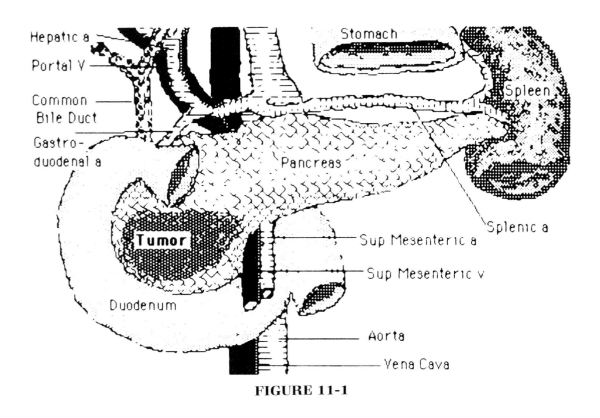

FIGURE 11-1

beyond the line of potential resection, making possible a decision as to resectability of the tumor or the alternative option of permanent interstitial implantation with I-125 seeds. Furthermore, it allows restoration of the continuity of the biliary, pancreatic, and gastrointestinal passages in as physiological a manner as possible. Brachytherapy is recommended for tumors localized to the pancreas or having minimal direct parapancreatic extension (**Fig. 11-1**). If regional nodal metastases (mainly celiac) are present and an implant of the primary site is feasible, a palliative interstitial implant may be done only in order to relieve pain. Supplementary external beam radiation may be considered in the latter case to increase the chance of local control. The presence of diffuse omental, peritoneal, or distant metastases is a contraindication to interstitial brachytherapy. Distant spread occurs mainly to the liver and lungs, with a lesser frequency to bones, the brain, and other anatomic sites.

Mobilization of the duodenum in lesions of the head of pancreas (Kocher's maneuver) will facilitate the determination of the posterior extent of the tumor (**Fig. 11-2**, left).

Once the tumor extent is determined, the three mutually perpendicular dimensions of the tumor are measured (Fig. 11-2, right).

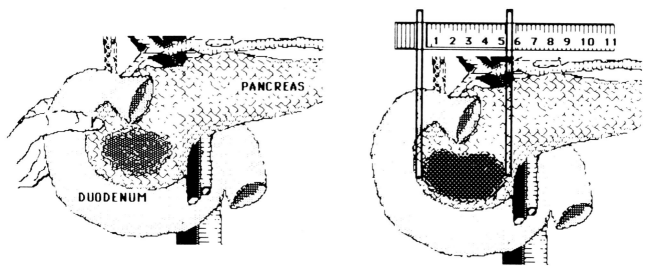

FIGURE 11-2

The length and width of the tumor are usually measured with the help of the caliper as shown in the previous figure. The anterioposterior dimension (depth) is measured by carefully placing a 15-cm implantation needle into the tumor. The length of the needle extending above the pancreas is measured with a stainless-steel ruler and this value is subtracted from the total length of the needle. The difference obtained indicates the depth of the tumor.

Prior to implantation, mobilization of the stomach and upward retraction will expose the anterior surface of the pancreas and facilitate the subsequent insertion of the implantation needles. The portal vein above the pancreas and the superior mesenteric vessels below the pancreas must be identified to avoid their injury.

The total activity to be implanted, the number of seeds, the spacing of needles and the spacing of seeds along each needle are determined by the New York–Memorial System of dosimetry using the permanent I-125 implantation nomograph. The predetermined number of needles are inserted into the pancreatic tumor until their tips can be sensed by the examining finger of the operator or his assistant placed behind the pancreas (**Fig. 11-3**, left). If bleeding occurs during the insertion of the needles secondary to puncture of small pancreatic vessels, the needle is retracted and pressure is applied using a sponge stick for 1 minute or longer if necessary. The needles should be placed parallel to each other as much as possible (Fig. 11-3, right). At the completion of the insertion, the operator should make sure that none of the needle tips have gone through the pancreas, which will result in loss of seeds into peritoneal cavity (**Fig. 11-4**, left). The special seed inserter is attached to one needle at a time with the aid of an Adson clamp and the I-125 seeds are inserted into the pancreatic tumor (Fig. 11-4, right). During the procedure, a careful record is kept of the number of I-125 seeds implanted, the activity per seed, and the spacing between seeds.

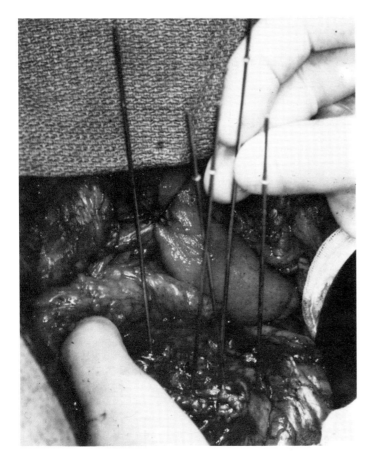

Needle placement

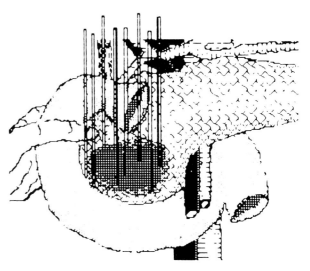

FIGURE 11-3

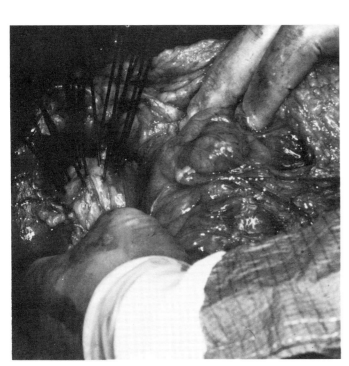

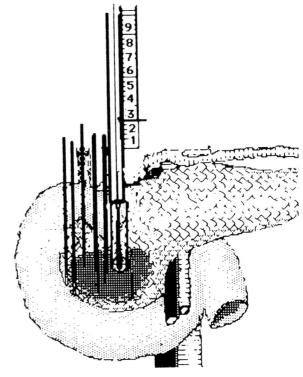

FIGURE 11-4

To avoid radiation damage to the adjacent stomach and duodenum, it is advisable to place the radioactive seeds at a distance of about 0.5 to 1.0 cm from the surface of the pancreas. Whenever feasible, at the end of the procedure a segment of the omentum is mobilized and positioned over the anterior surface of the implanted tumor in the pancreas to increase the distance between the implanted seeds and the bowel, and to prevent leakage of pancreatic fluid and, therefore, peritonitis.

A cholecystojejunostomy and/or gastrojejunostomy should be performed at the completion of brachytherapy in the presence of biliary or gastrointestinal obstruction. Small surgical hemoclips should be placed on the anterior surface of the pancreatic tumor to define and outline the region on future localization films for dosimetry evluation. The surgeon then closes the incision in the usual manner.

Localization radiographs are taken as soon as the patient becomes ambulatory, usually the third to fourth postoperative day.

Computerized dose calculations are displayed in orthogonal films (**Fig. 11-5**, left). If a CT scanner is available dosimetry can be displayed on appropriate CT transverse sections.

Follow-up localization radiographs are taken 2 to 6 months after the procedure to evaluate tumor regression by determining the position of the I-125 seeds (Fig. 11-5, right).

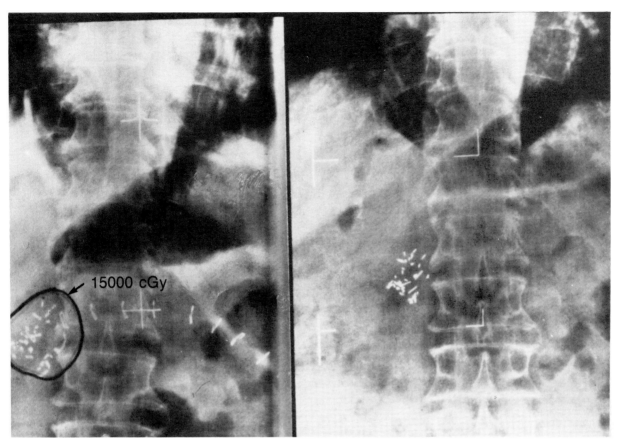

FIGURE 11-5

RESULTS

Intraoperative brachytherapy has received limited emphasis. Shipley and his coworkers have reported a mean survival of 11 months in 12 patients with localized cancer of the pancreas treated with I-125 interstitial brachytherapy.

During the period of 1975 to 1980 an analysis of 222 patients explored at Memorial Hospital showed that 33 patients were treated by brachytherapy. The in-hospital mortality was 3 percent in this group with no 30-day operative deaths. A median survival of 8 months was compared to biopsy alone of 3 months and resection for cure of 18 months. This showed a statistical improvement in favor of the patients who received brachytherapy.

In a more recent analysis, Manolatos et al. reviewed 96 patients with primary or recurrent unresectable pancreatic adenocarcinoma treated by brachytherapy at Memorial Hospital between 1974 and 1985. There were two groups of patients: 1) a group including all potentially curable patients with localized tumors, and 2) another group with patients who had regional or distant metastases. Twenty-four patients were alive at the time of the analysis. Median survival in group 1 was 38.5 weeks; in group 2, median survival was 20.7 weeks ($p = 0.006$).

Multivariate analysis demonstrated that the best survival was obtained in 1) patients who had tumors localized to the pancreas (T1–T3) with no evidence of regional or distant metastases (**Fig. 11-6**), and 2) patients with localized tumors (T1–T4) who received postoperative chemotherapy in addition to intraoperative brachytherapy. The survival in this category of patients was 52 weeks with chemotherapy versus 35 weeks without chemotherapy (**Fig. 11-7**). Sex, age, tumor site, treatment volume, and postoperative external radiation did not influence survival.

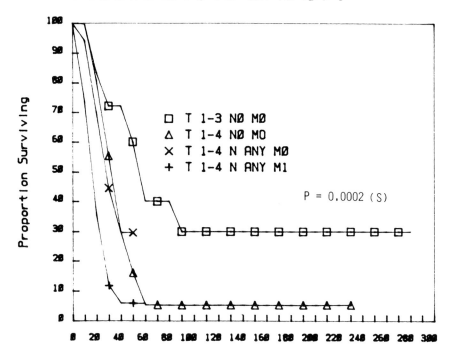

Pancreatic Carcinoma: T 1-3 NØ MØ VS
T 4 N Ø M Ø VS T 1-4 N ANY MØ VS M 1

□ T 1-3 NØ MØ
△ T 1-4 NØ MO
✕ T 1-4 N ANY MØ
+ T 1-4 N ANY M1

P = 0.0002 (S)

Weeks from Implant

FIGURE 11-6

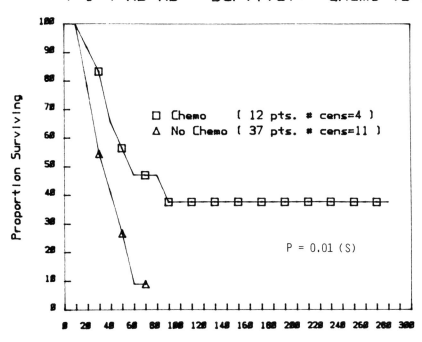

Pancreatic Carcinoma
T 1-4 NØ MØ - Survival: Chemo vs No Chemo

□ Chemo   (12 pts. # cens=4)
△ No Chemo (37 pts. # cens=11)

P = 0.01 (S)

Weeks from Implant

FIGURE 11-7

213

REFERENCES

1. Hilaris, B., Anderson, L. L., and Tokita, N. Interstitial implantation of pancreatic cancer. In: Vaeth, J. M. (ed.). *Frontiers of Radiation Oncology*. Basel, Switzerland: S. Karger, 1978, 12:62–71.

2. Shipley, W., Nardi, G., Cohen, A., and Ling, C. Iodine-125 implant and external beam irradiation in patients with localized pancreatic carcinoma. *Cancer* 45:709, 1980.

3. Barone, R. M. Treatment of carcinoma of the pancreas with radon seed implantation and intra-arterial infusion of 5-FUDR. *Surg Clin North Am* 55:117–128, 1975.

4. Morrow, M., Hilaris, B., and Brennan, M. F. Comparison and conventional surgical resection, radioactive implantation and bypass procedures for exocrine carcinoma of the pancreas, 1975–1980. *Ann Surg* 199:1–5, 1984.

5. Manolatos, S., Hilaris, B. S., Nori, D., Linares, L., Shiu, M. H., Anderson, L. L., and Brennan, M. Intraoperative brachytherapy in the management of locally advanced pancreatic cancer: identification of prognostic factors. In: *The Proceedings of the American Endocurietherapy Society Annual Meeting* 2(4):217, 1986.

6. Borgelt, B. Radiation therapy with either gold grain implant or neutron beam for unresectable adenocarcinoma of the pancreas. In: Cohn, I. (ed.). *Pancreatic Cancer New Directions in Therapeutic Management*. New York: Masson, 1980, pp. 55–63.

7. Whittington, R., Dobelbower, R., Borgelt, B., Rosato, F. E., Strubler, A., and Gelder, F. B. Combined 125-iodine implantation and precision high-dose radiotherapy in the treatment of unresectable pancreatic carcinoma. In: Cohn, I. (ed.). *Pancreatic Cancer New Directions in Therapeutic Management*. New York: Masson, 1980, pp. 31–42.

8. Brennan, M., Manolatos, S., Genest, P., and Hilaris, B. S. Brachytherapy in the management of pancreatic cancer. In: Hilaris, B. S., and Nori, D. (eds.). *Brachytherapy Oncology Update, 1984*. New York: Memorial Sloan-Kettering Cancer Center, 1984, pp. 29–41.

9. Shiu, M. H., Chang, J. Y., Brennan, M. F., Alfieri, A. A., and Hilaris, B. S. Mitomycin and concomittant iridium-192 brachytherapy of human pancreatic adenocarcinoma in the nude mouse. In: *The Proceedings of the American Endocurietherapy Society Annual Meeting* 2(4):218, 1986.

10. Dobelbower, R. R., Merrick, H. W., Ahuta, R. K., and Skeel, R. T. I-125 interstitial implant, precision high dose external beam therapy and 5fu for unresectable adenocarcinoma of the pancreas and extrahepatic biliary tree. *Cancer* 58:2185–2195, 1986.

11. Syed, N. A. M., Puthawala, A. A., and Neblett, D. L. Interstitial iodine-125 implant in the management of unresectable pancreatic carcinoma. *Cancer* 52:808–813, 1983.

CHAPTER 12

Brachytherapy for Cancer of the Prostate

Cancer of the prostate is the second most common cancer in males in the United States, representing about 20 percent of all cancer deaths in men. American blacks have the world's highest incidence, while the lowest incidence occurs in Asia. The incidence of prostatic carcinoma increases significantly with age, involving about one-half of the male population over the age of 70 years.

The most reliable signs for carcinoma on both ultrasound (particularly transrectally) and CT are a focal prostatic lesion and irregularity of the prostatic contour. The rectal examination, however, remains the most accurate and cost-effective test for detecting cancer of the prostate. The diagnosis is confirmed histologically by examination of a transurethral, transperineal or more commonly transrectal biopsy specimen of the prostatic lesion.

The lymph node drainage of the prostate follows the arterial supply. The principle route of lymphatic drainage is along the inferior vesicular artery from the so-called obturator nodes to the internal iliac (also called hypogastric) nodes (**Fig. 12-1**). Lesser nodes of prostatic drainage involve the external iliac, the presacral nodes, and the lateral sacral nodes. Prostatic cancer frequently metastasizes to pelvic lymph nodes before the clinical recognition of bone or visceral metastases. Because of the relative inaccuracy of pedal lymphangiography, sonography, and computerized tomography, pelvic lymphadenectomy is used by some as a staging modality.

Irradiation and/or surgery remain the standard treatments in early prostatic cancer. The respective roles of the two modalities have varied from time to time and from place to place. Interstitial brachytherapy alone or combined with external irradiation is another therapeutic option available for the management of cancer of the prostate.

Brachytherapy treatment planning is best done with CT because it can demonstrate local extension missed by other methods. CT is also ideal for showing the position of radioactive sources and the degree of tumor response after therapy (**Fig. 12-2**).

The two main methods of interstitial brachytherapy applied in cancer of the prostate are the permanent and the temporary interstitial techniques.

216

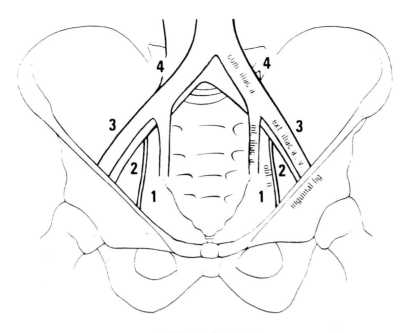

NODAL LEVELS

1. Medial to obturator nerve
2. Bet. ext. iliac vein & obturator nerve
3. Lat. & ant. to ext. iliac vessels
4. Above common iliac bifurcation

FIGURE 12-1

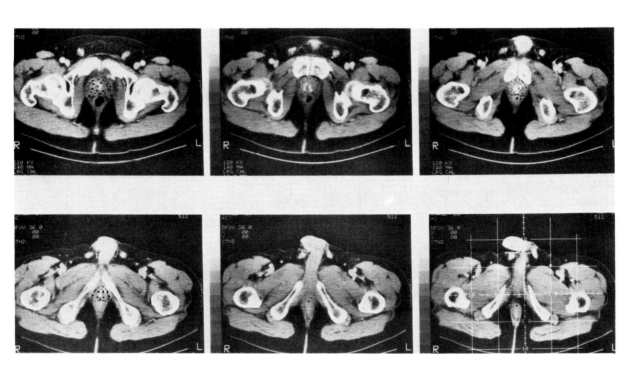

FIGURE 12-2

217

PERMANENT INTERSTITIAL BRACHYTHERAPY TECHNIQUE

Permanent implants can be performed by any one of the following approaches: 1) Through the perineum, above the anus, with the patient in the lithotomy position, recommended when a lymphadenectomy is not anticipated; 2) Through a suprapubic cystotomy with the needles placed directly in the prostate through the open bladder, an approach that has fallen in disrepute today; 3) Through a retropubic approach, which is recommended when a pelvic lymph node dissection is combined with the implant. More adequate manipulation is afforded by introducing a Foley catheter in the bladder and by inserting a finger into the rectum.

Retropubic Approach

The patient should be able to tolerate anesthesia and surgery with little or no risk. The patient is placed in the modified lithotomy position (**Fig. 12-3,** left upper) and prepared with an O'Connor's drape to allow a sterile rectal examination during the retropubic exploration. A preoperative examination under anesthesia and a cystoscopy is performed. A midline excision is then carried out, extending from the pubic symphysis to the umbilicus. At the end of the extraperitoneal staging lymphadenectomy the prostate is mobilized and inspected to insure adequate exposure for the radiation oncologist and to confirm that the tumor is confined within one lobe of the prostate. Surgical clips are placed on the prostate capsule at the midline, superiorly, inferiorly, and laterally to outline the prostatic gland (**Fig. 12-3,** right upper corner). This is an important step because it facilitates the measurement of the gland dimensions, outlines the urethral track, and allows identification of the prostate on subsequent localization radiographs. The entire prostate gland is considered as the target volume to be implanted. The depth (anterioposterior diameter) is measured by subtracing the protruding length of a needle from its total length of 15 cm (**Fig. 12-3,** middle left). The width and length are measured using a caliper, which is applied firmly on the gland, but without compressing it (**Fig. 12-3,** middle right). The permanent I-125 volume implant nomogram (see New York–Memorial system of dosimetry) is used to calculate the required number of I-125 seeds, the spacing between needles and seeds, and the required number of needles. The insertion of the needles begins at the superior medial margin of the prostate near the bladder base, in a row about 0.5 to 0.75 cm lateral to the urethra, to avoid puncturing it (**Fig. 12-3,** lower left). Using the precalculated spacing between needles, additional rows of needles are inserted into the prostate, until the entire gland is covered (**Fig. 12-3,** lower right). While the one lobe is implanted, the opposite side is packed with several 4 × 8-in gauzes to minimize the bleeding that inadvertently occurs when the needles puncture the abundant prostatic venous plexus.

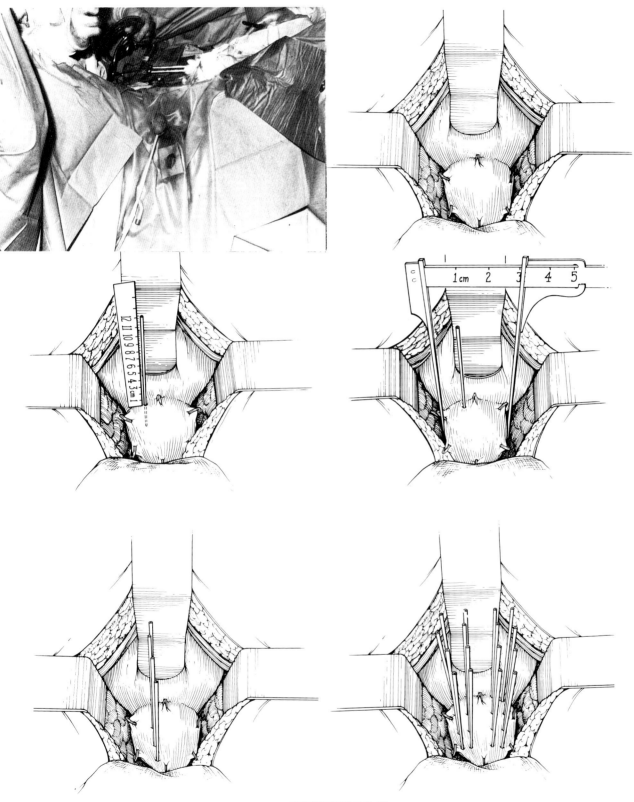

FIGURE 12-3

The needles should be inserted into the gland until their tips can be sensed in the rectum by the index finger of the operator or his assistant. Each needle is then retracted for a distance of 0.5 cm (the length of an I-125 seed). Precise depth of needle placement will ensure that the rectal wall is not violated, and there is space for the subsequent introduction of the radio-active seeds without risking the insertion of these seeds through the rectal musculature (**Fig. 12-4**, left upper). The special seed inserter applicator is attached to one needle at a time with the aid of an Adson clamp. The seeds are deposited into the prostatic tissue at precalculated spacings along the needle. Each needle is retracted after the seeds are deposited into the prostate and eventually removed from the gland. The same technique is repeated until all needles are removed.

The wound is drained with a Penrose drain, which is removed 2 to 3 days after the procedure. The implant dosimetry is done 24 to 48 hours after the brachytherapy procedure is performed and before the removal of the Foley catheter. Conventional dosimetry includes orthogonal anterior and lateral films or a stereo-shift method. The latter method is used when it is difficult to visualize the I-125 seeds on the lateral films. Computer calculations of dose distribution and isodose contours are superimposed and displayed preferably on CT cross sections (**Fig. 12-4,** right) or more conventionally on the orthogonal films (**Fig. 12-5,** left). A 3-D display might be used if a CT scan is not available (Fig. 12-5, right).

The tumor dose is reported as matched peripheral dose (MPD), matched integral dose (MID), and average dose (AD) (**Fig. 12-6**), as was discussed in more detail in Chap. 4.

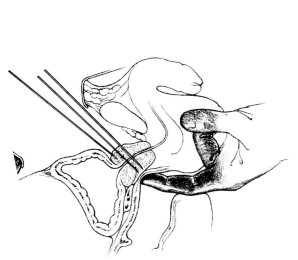 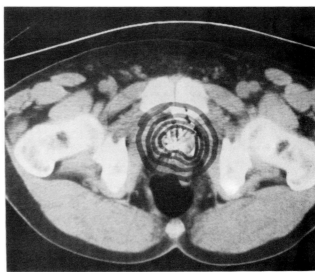

FIGURE 12-4

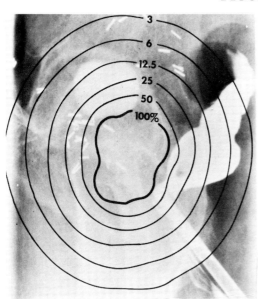 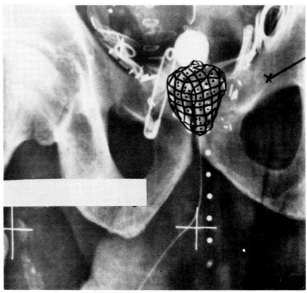

FIGURE 12-5

Evaluation Parameters

1 Matched peripheral dose corresponding to initial implant volume (MPD)	= _____ rad = _____ gray
2 Matched integral dose corresponding to initial implant volume (MID)	= _____ rad-kg = _____ joule
3 Average dose corresponding to initial implant volume (AD)	= _____ rad = _____ gray
4 Net integral dose outside implant, for dose ⩾ 80 gray (NID)	= _____ rad-kg = _____ joule

Minimum, Integral and Average Dose within Computed Volume

Minimum dose (rad)	40	80	120	160	200	240	280	320
Computed volume (cm³)								
Integral dose (joule)								
Average dose (gray)								

1 gray = 100 rad = 1 joule/kg

revised Jan 1977

15 - 1

FIGURE 12-6

Percutaneous Perineal Approach

All patients undergo a pretreatment CT scan of the pelvis with a rectal obturator and a template in place (**Fig. 12-7**); thin 5-mm sections are taken through the area of interest. CT allows tumor volume calculations with great precision, determination of the number of required seeds and their distribution within the prostate, as well as generation of preliminary iso-dose contours.

The actual procedure is performed 2 to 3 days later, usually under sedation and epidural nerve block. The rectal obturator is reintroduced in the patient's rectum and the template used for the planning is attached to the obturator and pushed against the perineum. It is immobilized at this position with a thumbscrew. The calculated number of needles is inserted through the template holes, under direct fluoroscopic control (anterio-posterior and lateral), advanced through the perineum, and pushed to the precalculated depth. The point of entry of each needle is the previously placed reference mark on the template. The position of each needle within the tumor should be checked fluoroscopically to correspond to the precalculated one (**Fig. 12-8**).

At the completion of the insertion of all needles, radioactive I-125 seeds are loaded in the needles, which are then removed. Plastic marks are placed on the skin over the implanted area for dosimetry purpose and orthogonal radiographs (**Fig. 12-9,** left) and CT scans similar to the ones taken prior to the implantation are repeated for the final dosimetry. If stable, the patient could be discharged home the following day. The final dosimetry is displayed either superimposed to an orthogonal radiograph (Fig. 12-9, right) or to a scan.

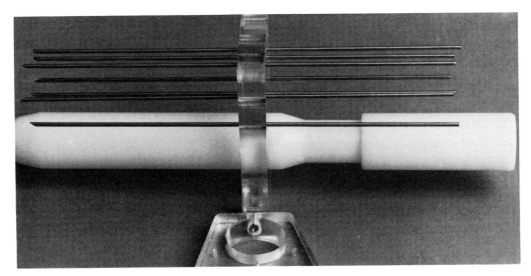

FIGURE 12-7

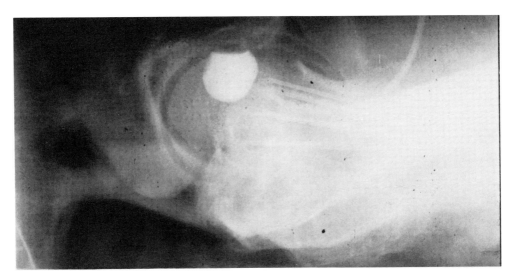

FIGURE 12-8

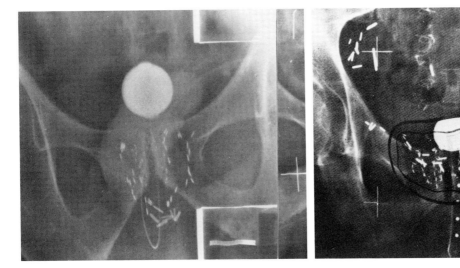

FIGURE 12-9

TEMPORARY PERINEAL INTERSTITIAL BRACHYTHERAPY TECHNIQUE

This technique is similar to the one described previously for permanent perineal implantation. It utilizes either commercially available templates, i.e., Syed (**Fig. 12-10**), Martinez et al., or custom-made perineal templates (Memorial technique) to guide the insertion of needles into the prostate and hold them in place.

The procedure is done under general anesthesia with the patient in a modified lithotomy position and a Foley catheter inserted into the bladder. Needles are inserted transperineally into the prostate in the predetermined by the CT plan positions. The template is fixed to the perineum by "00" silk suture (**Fig. 12-11**).

The final dosimetric calculations are done on the basis of post-implantation orthogonal x-ray localization films with dummy sources in place (**Fig. 12-12**). If a CT scanner is available, CT cuts at a distance of 0.5 to 1 cm are also taken.

Computerized isodose contours are obtained, and the appropriate dose rate covering all of the designated target area is selected. Relatively homogeneous dose distribution is obtained either by differential unloading of the radioactive Ir-192 or I-125 seeds or by using different activity seeds. Standardized loadings should be avoided as much as possible because they tend either to overirradiate normal tissues or to underirradiate the target volume. Loading and unloading of the sources is performed in the conventional manner as described in Chap. 3.

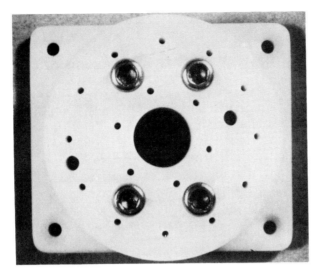

FIGURE 12-10

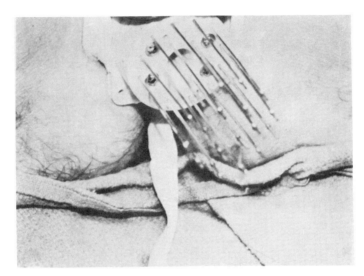

FIGURE 12-11

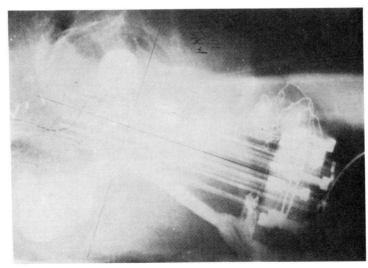

FIGURE 12-12

Percutaneous Implantation with Transrectal Ultrasound Guidance

Recent advances in ultrasound technology have made possible the development of a transrectal ultrasound unit (Bruel & Kjar, Denmark), which permits simple and accurate needle guidance for percutaneous interstitial brachytherapy. A high-resolution display image provides great detail of the prostate. A probe-stepping unit allows accurate volume determinations of the prostatic gland.

The brachytherapy procedure is performed under spinal anesthesia with the patient in a modified lithotomy position. A template grid attached to the unit improves the accuracy of the procedure (**Fig. 12-13**).

Several modifications of the existing equipment have been devised to improve the stability of the apparatus and the accuracy of the implant.

An ultrasound tumor volume and dose evaluation after implantation is shown in **Fig. 12-14**.

Transrectal scanning has the potential of excellent tumor localization, prostate volume determination, improved brachytherapy planning, and accurate brachytherapy dose evaluation.

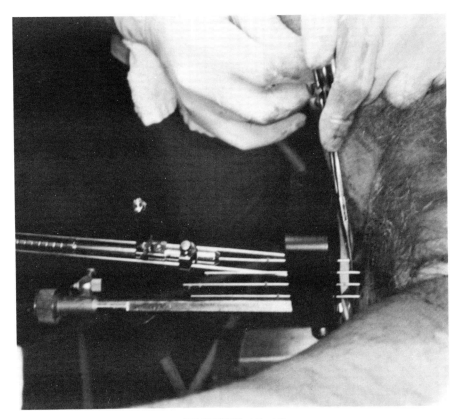

FIGURE 12-13

CODE	LEVEL	CGy
1	25.0	4000
2	50.0	2000
3	75.0	12000
4	100.0	16000
5	150.0	24000
6	200.0	32000

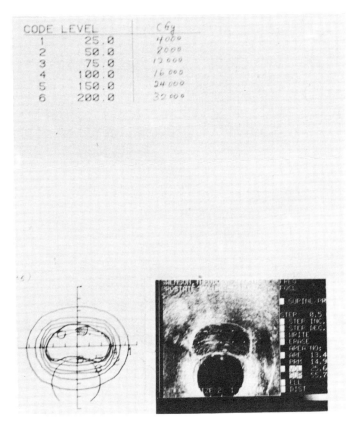

FIGURE 12-14

RESULTS

Beginning in 1970, selected patients with stage B or small C prostatic cancer have been treated at Memorial Sloan-Kettering Cancer Center by pelvic lymph node dissection and interstitial I-125 brachytherapy. The procedure had a low morbidity and mortality (4 deaths in 1100 patients = 0.36 percent), and has been associated with more than 90 percent preservation of sexual potency.

Survival rates of 160 patients followed for at least 10 years for B_1, B_2, B_3, and C lesions with negative nodes were approximately 72 percent, 66 percent, 58 percent, and 50 percent, respectively. Local failures with or without distant metastases were evident in approximately 20 percent of B_1 lesions and 40 percent of B_2, B_3, and C lesions.

Similar results were reported by Shipley et al. for patients treated at Massachusetts General Hospital from 1973 to 1981 with a minimum follow up of 5 years. Among 370 patients treated during the preceding period, 51 patients received 1050 cGy preoperative external beam radiation followed by I-125 brachytherapy. The remaining patients were treated with external pelvic radiation and a boost to the primary given either by photons (259 patients) or by protons (60 patients). No significant difference was observed in survival or local control among the 3 groups.

In 1986, Morton et al. reported a retrospective comparison of 106 patients treated by I-125 implantation and 73 patients treated by external beam radiation. There was no difference either in the disease-free 5-year survival rate (75 percent) or in the absolute local tumor-control rate (85 to 88 percent) for stage B patients, regardless of treatment, confirming the value of brachytherapy for early cancer of the prostate.

More recently (1986) Deblasio et al. analyzed the results of treatment of 99 patients treated at Memorial Sloan-Kettering Cancer Center in 1981 and demonstrated that high local tumor control rate can be expected with the full I-125 implant dose of 16,000 cGy (**Fig. 12-15**). The upper part of this figure shows the local control according to the stage; the lower part shows the local control according to the lymph node status and the histological grade.

LOCAL CONTROL BY STAGE

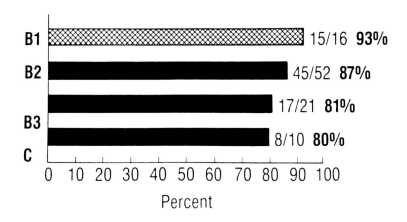

LOCAL CONTROL

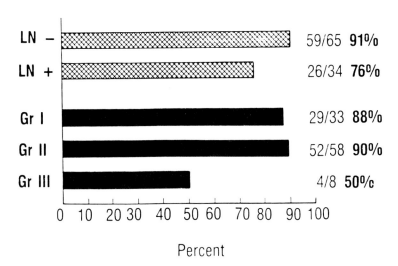

FIGURE 12-15

REFERENCES

1. Pasteau, O., and Degrais, A. The radium treatment of cancer of the prostate. *Arch. Roentgen Ray* 28:396–410, 1913–1914.

2. Young, H. H. The use of radium in cancer of the prostate and bladder. *JAMA* 68:1174, 1917.

3. Barringer, B. S. Radium in the treatment of carcinoma of the bladder and prostate. *JAMA* 68:1227–1230, 1917.

4. Batata, M. A., Hilaris, B. S., Chu, F. C. H., Whitmore, W. F., Song, H. S., Kim, Y., Horowitz, B., and Song, K. S. Radiation therapy in adenocarcinoma of the prostate with pelvic lymph node involvement on lymphadenectomy. *Int J Radiat Oncol Biol Phys* 6:149–153, 1980.

5. Kumar, P. P., Good, R. R., Rainbolt, C., Epstein, B. E., Chu, W. K., Jones, E. O., Cascione, C. J., and Hussain, M. B. Low morbidity following transperineal percutaneous template technique for permanent iodine-125 endocurietherapy of prostate cancer. *Endocuriether Hyperthermia Oncol* 2:119–126, 1986.

6. Holm, H. H., Stryer, I., Hansen, H., et al. Ultrasonically guided percutaneous interstitial implantation of iodine-125 seeds in cancer therapy. *Br J Radiol* 54:665–670, 1981.

7. Kim, R. Y., Brascho, D. J., and Wilson, A. E. Use of ultrasound scan in prostatic I-125 implantation. *Int J Radiat Oncol Biol Phys* 10:1971–1973, 1984.

8. Brindle, J. S., Benson, R. C., Martinez, A., Edmundson, G. K., Zincke, H., and Utz, D. C. Acute toxicity and preliminary therapeutic results of pelvic lymphadenectomy combined with transperineal interstitial implantation of Ir-192 and external beam radiotherapy for locally advanced prostate cancer. *Urology* 25:233–238, 1985.

9. Martinez, A., Edmundson, G. K., Cox, R. S., Guuderson, L. L., and Howes, A. E. Combination of external beam irradiation and multiple-site perineal applicator (MUPIT) for treatment of locally advanced or recurrent prostate, anorectal, and gynecologic malignancies. *Int J Radiat Oncol Bio Phys* 11:391–393, 1985.

10. Syed, A. M. N., Puthawala, A., Tarsey, L. A., Schanberg, A. M.: Temporary Ir-192 implantation in the management of carcinoma of the prostate. In: Hilaris, B. S., Batata, M., (eds.), *Brachytherapy Oncology*. New York: Memorial Sloan-Kettering Cancer Center, 1983.

11. Blasko, J. C., Ragde, H., and Schumacher, D. Transperineal iodine-125 implantation with transrectal ultrasound guidance for prostatic carcinoma (abstr.) *Endocuriether Hyperthermia Oncol* 2:209, 1986.

12. Morton, J. D., Harrison, L. B., and Peschel, R. E. Prostatic cancer therapy: comparison of external-beam radiation and I-125 seed implantation treatment of stages B and C neoplasms. *Radiology* 159:249–252, 1986.

13. Shipley, W. U., Coachman, N. M., McNulty, P. A., Healy, E. A., Elman, A. J., Proute, G. R., Heney, N. M., Althausen, A. F., and Suit, H. D. Radiation therapy of men with localized prostatic carcinoma: the Massachusetts General Hospital experience. Abstract presented at NIH Consensus Development Conference on Management of Clinically Localized Prostate Cancer, pp. 51–54, June 15–17, 1987.

CHAPTER 13

Brachytherapy
in
Cancer of the Bladder

Carcinoma of the urinary bladder accounts for approximately 2 percent of all malignant tumors. Traditionally, management of patients with carcinoma of the bladder has been the responsibility of the urologic surgeon. Now, however, proper management requires the concerted effort of a team approach, with involvement from the radiotherapist and medical oncologist, as well as the urologist. The increased incidence of bladder cancer and the rising mortality from bladder cancer underscore the need for effective combination treatment programs for all stages of disease in order to reduce recurrences and improve survival rates.

Carcinoma in situ or superficial transitional cell carcinoma traditionally has been treated with transurethral resection (TUR) and fulguration, or with chemotherapeutic agents. External irradiation has been used in the treatment of a few of these patients with unsatisfactory results. Partial resection, cystectomy, radical radiation, and a combination of radiotherapy and cystectomy are being used for invasive disease (B–C or T2–T3). The disappointing long-term survival statistics in patients with deeply invasive tumors undergoing radical cystectomy or radiotherapy have led to the introduction of the combined approach using planned, preoperative irradiation. Despite the active and popular use of preoperative ERT and radical cystectomy by the majority of centers over the past 15 to 20 years, however, no clear definite benefit of the adjuvant ERT has been identified.

Brachytherapy for bladder tumors was originally described by Barringer at Memorial Hospital and consisted of the introduction of a radium capsule through the cystoscope. Barringer later expanded this treatment by using

232

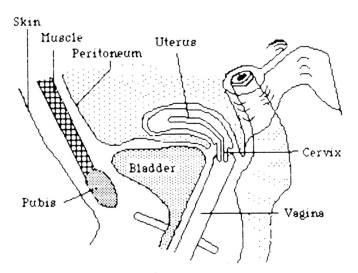

FIGURE 13-1

radon seeds implanted in and around the tumor. Various other brachytherapy approaches have been used, i.e., endoscopic, perineal, vaginal, and through a suprapubic cystotomy. All these efforts set the stage for the brachytherapy approach that proved so successful in Rotterdam and more recently in Paris.

Patients selected for curative brachytherapy should have early stage (T1, T2), small tumors less than 5 cm in diameter, unifocal, located in the dome or slightly extended to the trigone of the bladder.

Noninvasive delineation of the tumor volume is obtained by CT scan, intravenous pyelography, when indicated, and cystoscopy under anesthesia. Final tumor delineation is frequently determined at the time of surgery. The bladder is a retropubic and extraperitoneal organ; its relationship to other pelvic organs is shown in **Fig. 13-1** (female) and in **Fig. 13-2** (male).

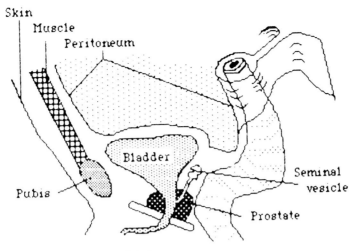

FIGURE 13-2

Temporary Interstitial Brachytherapy Suture Technique

This afterloading technique has been described previously in Chap. 3. It is performed under general anesthesia following a suprapubic cystotomy and opening of the bladder distant to the tumor site. The usual plan is to implant afterloading catheters 1 cm apart to cover the tumor and a short distance around. The thin end of the nylon catheter (leader) is threaded through the eye of a surgical curved needle, sutured through the bladder wall about 2 cm superior to the tumor, pushed through the bladder wall, and exiting about 2 cm below the tumor. Other tubes are introduced in the same way parallel with the first one and spaced according to the guidelines of the New York system of dosimetry using the single-plane Ir-192 nomogram. When the introduction of all nylon tubes is finished, they are brought out of the abdomen, away from the incision. This is usually done through straight or curved needles inserted percutaneously above the pubic symphysis (**Fig. 13-3**a); both the needle and the thin leader of each nylon tube are pulled and brought out (Fig. 13-3b). The needle is then removed and the catheter is cut 2 to 3 cm distance from the skin (Fig. 13-3c).

The catheters are fixed on the skin of the anterior abdominal wall with the usual plastic hemisphere and metal button which is then sutured on the skin (**Fig. 13-4**).

If a partial cystectomy has been performed the steps of implantation are similar, but only two catheters are used; one on either side of the bladder incision, which is then closed.

Localization orthogonal radiographs are taken the same day or the day following the insertion of the afterloading catheters and computerized dosimetric calculations are performed.

The loading of the radioactive Ir-192 sources is performed 5 to 6 days after surgery in the patient's room.

The Ir-192 sources first and the nylon tubes immediately afterward are removed under aseptic conditions at the completion of the treatment without reopening the bladder. After treatment, a mucosal erythematous reaction develops within the bladder mucosa, corresponding to the implanted region, which clears slowly within 6 to 10 weeks.

Target Volume. Includes the tumor volume (the tumor bed, if debulking was performed) and a margin of at least 1 to 2 cm around it.

Target Dose. Consists of 6000 cGy, if the histological margins of resection are positive; 4500 cGy, if the margins are negative.

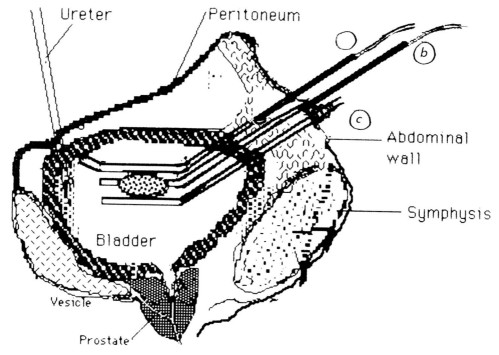

FIGURE 13-3

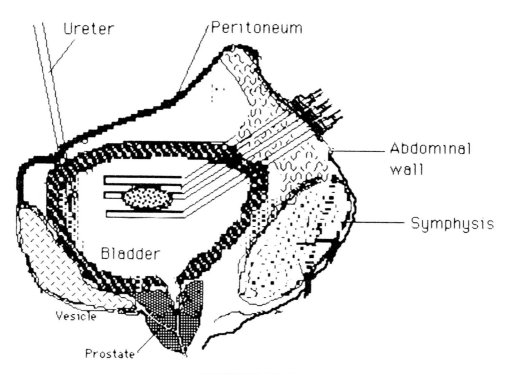

FIGURE 13-4

Intracavitary Brachytherapy Technique

Intracavitary techniques are used to deliver a boost dose to the primary tumor after external beam radiation and for the treatment of recurrences after radiation. They have very limited application.

The first technique was described by Barringer in 1917, who used it at Memorial hospital. A Ra-226 source was introduced through the urethra with the help of a cystoscope and was left in position for 6 to 8 hours.

A modification of this technique was used by Friedman and Lewis at the Walter Reed Hospital in the 1940s. A Ra-226, Rn-222, or Co-60 source was centrally positioned in the bladder via a suprapubic cystotomy.

More recently, an intracavitary technique was described by Kumar et al, using a miniaturized Cs-137 source. This treatment method is combined with external pelvic radiation, which consists initially of 4000 cGy in 5 weeks using opposing fields, followed by a boost 2000 cGy in 2.5 weeks with a rotational technique. The intracavitary source is introduced via a Foley catheter, following appropriate localization and dosimetric studies using a dummy source. The final position of the Cs-137 source is again checked by orthogonal films (**Fig. 13-5**). Computed isodose contours are then superimposed on the orthogonal films or a CT scan slice of the pelvis (**Fig. 13-6**) to display the dose distribution.

Similar techniques may be used with remote afterloading of the radioactive sources, using either low dose rate or high dose rate brachytherapy.

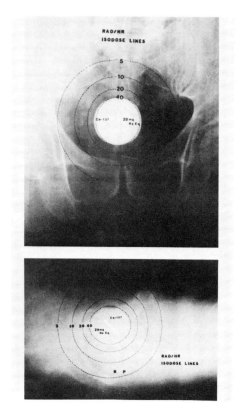

FIGURE 13-5

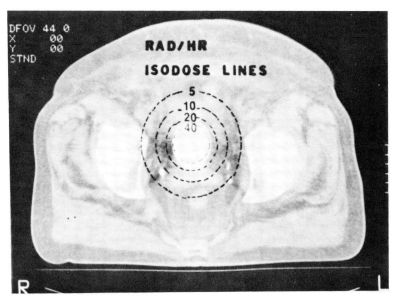

FIGURE 13-6

RESULTS

At the Rotterdam Radiotherapy Institute, the Netherlands, a prospective randomized study of TUR alone versus TUR followed by implantation of radium needles in the bladder through a suprapubic route has resulted in a higher tumor control in the combined treatment group. Seventy-five percent of the TUR cases had at least one bladder relapse, but only 18 percent of the radium patients had the same problem. Of the patients treated with TUR alone, 25 percent had to undergo 4 to 10 subsequent TUR resections for local recurrence, in contrast to only 3 percent of the patients who were treated with intracavitary radium.

Over the past decade many institutions have reported that modern megavoltage irradiation can be curative, but only for a minority of patients with muscle-invading primary carcinoma of the bladder. The overall 5-year survival rates have been low for patients with clinical stages B2 and C (17 to 38 percent). Van der Werf-Messing, however, reported a 60-percent 5- and 10-year survival in similar stage patients treated by external irradiation combined with intravesical radium implantation.

Mazeron and others have recently reported preliminary encouraging results in 55 patients treated with a combination of preoperative external pelvic radiation, limited partial cystectomy, and Ir-192 interstitial brachytherapy. Thirty-seven patients (67 percent) were alive at 5 years without evidence of disease.

The Rotterdam Radiotherapy Institute's experience, the largest one with interstitial brachytherapy, is summarized in **Table 13-1.**

TABLE 13-1. Rotterdam Radiotherapy Institute Experience

Stage	Patients at Risk	Treatment	5-Year Survial (%)
T1NXMO	195	Radium	80 (better than ERT* alone)
T2NXMO	328	External rad & radium+	75 (better than ERT* alone)
T3NXMO	41	External rad & radium 55%‡	74 (equal to preop ERT* and cystectomy)

* = external pelvic radiation.

+ = 350 cGy × 3 followed by full radium dose.

‡ = 4000 cGy ERT followed by 55 percent of the full radium dose.

REFERENCES

1. Barringer, B. S. Discussion of treatment of cancer of the bladder and prostate. In: Janeway, H. H. *Radium Therapy in Cancer at the Memorial Hospital, New York (First Report: 1915–1916)*. New York: Paul B. Hoeber, 1917.

2. Barringer, B. S. Technique of suprapubic implantation of radon seeds in bladder carcinoma. *Surg Gynecol Obstet* 55:487–489, 1932.

3. Darget, R. La radiumtherapie des tumeurs vesicales. *Bull Soc franc d'Urol*, 1931, pp. 171–173.

4. Lenz, M., Cahill, G. F., Melicow, M. M., and Donlan, C. P. Treatment of cancer of bladder by radium needles. *Am J Roentgenol* 58:486–491, 1947.

5. Emmett, J. L., and Winterringer, J. R. Experience with implantation of radon seeds for bladder tumors: comparison of results with other forms of treatment. *J Urol* 73:502–515, 1955.

6. Bloom, H. J. Treatment of carcinoma of the bladder: a symposium. 1. Treatment by interstitial irradiation using tantalum 182 wire. *Br J Radiol* 33:471–479, 1960.

7. Durrant, K. R., and Laing, A. H. Treatment of multiple superficial papillary tumors of the bladder by intracavity yttrium-90. *J Urol* 113:480, 1975.

8. Ellis, F. Cancer of the bladder. In: Hilaris, B. S. (ed.). *Handbook of Interstitial Brachytherapy*. Acton, Mass.: Publishing Sciences Group, 1975, pp. 241–250.

9. van der Werf-Messing, B., and Hop, W. C. J. Carcinoma of the urinary bladder (category T1NXM0) treated either by radium implant or by transurethral resection only. *Int J Radiat Oncol Biol Phys* 7:299–303, 1981.

10. Whitmore, W. F., and Prout, G. R., III, Jr. Discouraging results of high dose external beam radiation therapy in low stage (O and A) bladder cancer. *J Urol* 127:902–905, 1982.

11. van der Werf-Messing, B. H. P., Menon, R. S., and Hop, W. C. J. Interstitial radiotherapy of carcinoma of the bladder at the Rotterdam Radiotherapy Institute (RRTI). In: *Progress and Controversies in Oncological Urology*, Kurth K. H., Debruyne, F. M. J., Schroeder, F. H., Splinter, T. A. W., and Wagener, T. D. J. (eds.). New York: Alan R. Liss, 1984, pp. 297–310.

12. Mazeron, J. J., Marinello, G., Leung, S., LeBourgeois, J. P., Abbou, C. C., Auvert, J., and Pierquin, B. Treatment of bladder tumors by iridium 192 implantation. The Creteil technique. *Radiother Oncol* 1985, pp. 111–119.

13. Kumar, P. P., and Good, R. R. Afterloading of intracavitary endocurietherapy for carcinoma of the bladder using cesium-137 mini-sources. *Endocuriether Hyperthermia Oncol* 3:11–17, 1987.

14. van der Werf-Messing, B. H. P. Interstitial radiation therapy of carcinoma of the urinary bladder. *Endocuriether Hyperthermia Oncol* 2:67–76, 1986.

CHAPTER 14

Brachytherapy in Cancer of the Cervix

CANCER OF THE UTERINE CERVIX

The most common primary tumor in the uterine cervix is squamous cell carcinoma (95 percent), followed by adenocarcinoma, adenoacanthoma, and undifferentiated tumors, making up the remaining 5 percent. Clinically, cervical tumors may be exophytic, endophytic, or ulcerative. The endophytic tumors constitute the type characterized clinically as *barrel-shaped.*

Cancer of the uterine cervix initially spreads by direct invasion and/or lymphatic metastases. The initial sites of lymph node metastases are the obturator nodes and the nodes at the level of the bifurcation of the internal and external iliacs (**Fig. 14-1**).

Although the focus of this chapter is brachytherapy, radiation therapy, for all but very early stage cancer of the cervix, involves external beam as well, because the aim is to treat both the primary tumor and the regional pelvic nodes. As a rule the external beam proportion of total dose increases with stage of the disease.

Out treatment policy governing the two modalities as a function of stage is shown in **Table 14-1.**

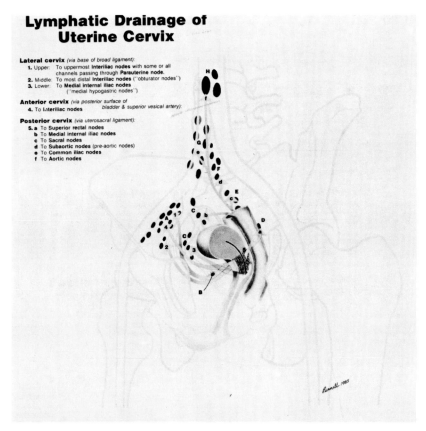

Lymphatic Drainage of Uterine Cervix

Lateral cervix *(via base of broad ligament):*
1. Upper: To uppermost **Interiliac** nodes with some or all channels passing through **Parauterine** node.
2. Middle: To most distal **Interiliac** nodes ("obturator nodes")
3. Lower: To **Medial internal iliac** nodes ("medial hypogastric nodes")

Anterior cervix *(via posterior surface of bladder & superior vesical artery):*
4. To **Interiliac** nodes

Posterior cervix *(via uterosacral ligament):*
5. a To **Superior rectal** nodes
   b To **Medial internal iliac** nodes
   c To **Sacral** nodes
   d To **Subaortic** nodes (pre-aortic nodes)
   e To **Common iliac** nodes
   f To **Aortic** nodes

FIGURE 14-1

TABLE 14-1

Stage	External Whole-Pelvis (Rads)	Interval (Weeks)	Intracavitary (Dose to Reference Point in Rads)	Other Standard Treatments
IA	—	—	3000–3 weeks–3000	Simple hysterectomy
IB	a	2	2500–2 weeks–2500	Radical hysterectomy with bilateral pelvic lymphadenectomy
IIA	4000/4 weeks			
IIB	5000/5 weeks Use central shield after 4000 rads	2	2500–2 weeks–2500	—
IIIA	b 5000/5 weeks Use central shield after 4000 rads	2	2500–2 weeks–2500	—
IIIB	6000/6 weeks and central shield after 4000 rads	2–3	4000	—
IV	6500/6.5 weeks and central shield after 4000 rads	2–3	Possibly one application of 3000 rads	—

[a]Extend the treatments to 5000 rads in 5 weeks for barrel-shaped lesions and also consider simple abdominal hysterectomy after external pelvic radiation and one intracavitary application. Similar treatment is also suggested when disease extends into the endometrial cavity.

[b]Field lengthened to include all disease with 2- to 3-cm margin. External pelvic radiation should be given with four-field technique on a linear accelerator with appropriate small bowel, rectal, and bladder shields in the lateral beam. Computerized dose distribution should be performed for all intracavitary procedures to document rectal and bladder doses.

Intracavitary Cervix Irradiation

The most common methods of intracavitary irradiation have been patterned after the Manchester system, with a treatment-dose reference point defined in a manner similar to the definition of the Manchester point A. The definitions developed at Memorial Hospital for both tumor and normal tissue points, and the associated dose objectives for stages Ib and II cervix cancer, are listed in **Table 14-2.** Tolerance points are those for which the target dose is stated as an upper limit. The target dose rate at the reference point is 60 cGy/hour. We strongly recommend that the reader consults, in addition, chapter 5 for more extensive discussion of intracavitary planning and evaluation.

The cervix intracavitary technique is illustrated by the Henschke technique described in Chap. 3. The application is usually performed under general anesthesia, although it can be done under an epidural or spinal block. The patient is placed in the lithotomy position. It should be emphasized that an examination and extensive evaluation of the extent of the disease should take place prior to the brachytherapy procedure, to allow an accurate staging. The examination includes a proctosigmoidoscopy and cystoscopy to evaluate any abnormalities. When possible, this examination should be done jointly by the gynecologist and the radiation oncologist. Instruments for probing, dilating, and inserting the Henschke applicator are shown in **Fig. 14-2** (left).

The first step of the technique is the identification of the cervix, which is grasped with a uterine tenaculum to prevent its movement (Fig. 14-2, right).

The endometrial canal is sounded to determine its length and position (**Fig. 14-3,** left), and the cervix is dilated with a Haynes (# 16) dilator (Fig. 14-3, right).

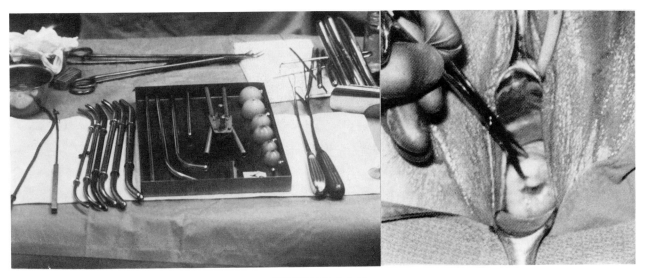

FIGURE 14-2

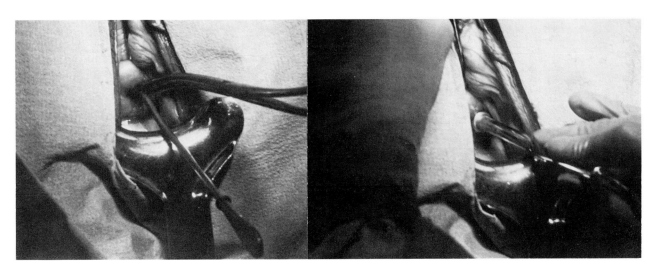

FIGURE 14-3

TABLE 14-2. Dose Specification for Cervix Cancer Intracavitary
Treatments at Memorial Hospital

Point	Location	Target Dose (cGy)
Reference	2 cm superior, 2 cm lateral from cervical os	2500
Cervix	1 cm superior, 1 cm lateral from cervical os	5000
Uterus	1 cm inferior, 2 cm lateral from tandem tip	2100
Vagina	Lateral surface of ovoid	2500
Rectum	5 probe points 1 cm apart	<1200
Sigmoid	Midway between tandem tip and promontorium	<1200
Bladder	Center of catheter balloon	<1500

An assembled applicator, prior to insertion, is shown in **Fig. 14-4.**

A #16 gauge Foley catheter, with a 10 mL balloon, is inserted into the bladder. The balloon is filled with 1 mL of radiopaque material and 9 mL of normal saline. At this point a tandem with a curvature approximating that of the endometrial canal is selected. The cervical flange is adjusted to provide a tandem slightly less than the measured length of the uterine canal (**Fig. 14-5,** left). Two surgical clips are placed on the outer surface of the cervix for subsequent radiographic localization. The intrauterine tandem, with the adjusted flange set at the selected tandem length, is introduced into the uterine canal (Fig. 14-5, right).

An ovoid size is selected that will allow easy insertion and separation. These colpostats are attached to the central tandem of the applicator (**Fig. 14-6,** left). Each colpostat is adjusted in such a way that its center is at the level of the cervical flange. The colpostats are spread as far apart as possible. The completed insertion of the assembled applicator is shown in Fig. 14-6, right.

The vagina is packed with a 22-inch gauze soaked in Betadine and pushed between the posterior wall of the vagina and the colpostats. The same is repeated anteriorly.

The applicator is secured with a mattress suture through the labia majora, sewn above the applicator. The adequacy of packing is checked by rectal examination. If the colpostats are felt, the posterior packing is inadequate, and should be removed and reinserted. The applicator is further secured by a T-shaped male binder. A rectal tube is inserted into the rectum, for subsequent localization radiographs, and secured on the skin by tape.

The insertion and removal of the radioactive sources is performed in the patient's room. After the removal of the active sources, the Foley catheter is deflated; the skin suture and the vaginal packing are then removed. Colpostat spreading is released and the applicator is rotated 45 degrees and pulled out gently. The patient is examined for bleeding, lacerations, and so forth. The parts of the applicator are accounted for to make sure that everything has been removed.

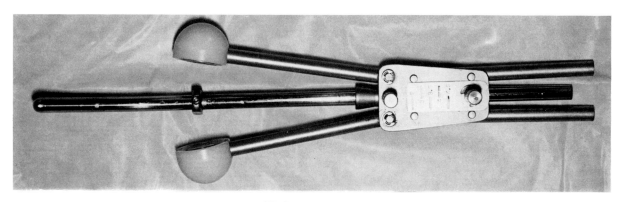

FIGURE 14-4

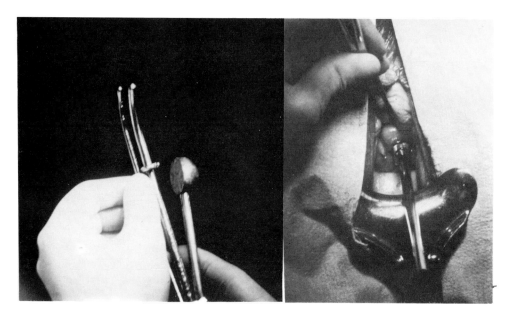

FIGURE 14-5

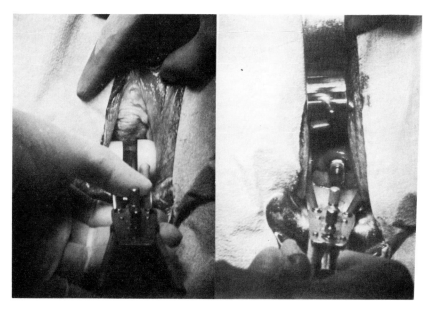

FIGURE 14-6

Template Techniques

Adequate dose distribution with intracavitary applicators is possible for patients with early stage cancer of the cervix and in those patients with relatively advanced disease that has responded well to initial external beam radiation. In patients with extensive disease involving the parametria and vagina, however, conventional intracavitary applications do not provide an adequate dose distribution to the target volume without excessive irradiation of the rectum and bladder. Furthermore, in patients where the tandem cannot be used (even in early stage disease), such as carcinoma of the cervical stump, obliterated canal due to fibrosis or tumor, and so forth, a satisfactory dose distribution with intravaginal colpostats alone cannot in general be achieved.

Template techniques are used to improve the homogeneity of pelvic radiation by adding an interstitial component. The total dose prescribed with these procedures depends on the dose already delivered with external beam, as well as the extent of the disease and the dose to the critical normal tissues, i.e., rectum and bladder.

Insertion of Syed–Neblett Template

All template insertions are performed under general anesthesia following a pelvic examination to determine the extent of the disease and the response to external beam irradiation. The assembled template is shown in **Fig. 14-7.**

The patient's preparation, the uterus sounding, the endocervical canal's dilatation, and the insertion of the central tandem are identical to a cervix intracavitary application. A guide needle is inserted into the 6 o'clock groove on the obturator and implanted into the posterior lip of the cervix. The vaginal obturator is then introduced, with the inferior portion of the tandem exiting through its central opening (**Fig. 14-8,** left). The length of the tandem extending beyond the end of the vaginal obstructor is measured. The central slit on the tandem serves to indicate the orientation of the tandem. The template is guided over the obturator against the perineum (Fig. 14-8, right) and secured to the perineum with a 1-0 silk suture and to the vaginal obturator by tightening the thumbscrew (**Fig. 14-9,** left). A Foley catheter is inserted and its balloon is inflated with 10 mL of Renografin (Squibb Diagnostics, A Division of E. R. Squibb & Sons, New Brunswick, NJ 08903). The needles (usually 20-cm long) closest to the anterior rectal wall are inserted first. Their position is checked by rectal examination to assure that they are not in the rectum. The remaining needles are then inserted. The paracervical or parametrial needles should not be pushed more than 3 to 4 cm beyond the level of the external os. The depth of insertion can be determined from the length of each needle protruding outside the template (Fig. 14-9, right).

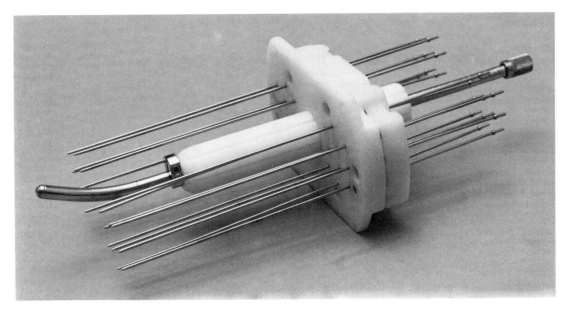

FIGURE 14-7

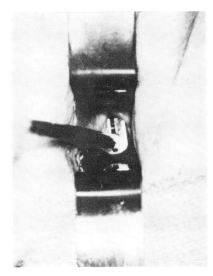
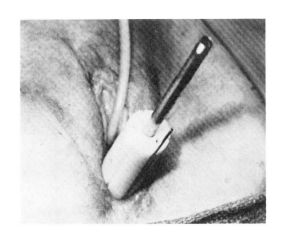

FIGURE 14-8

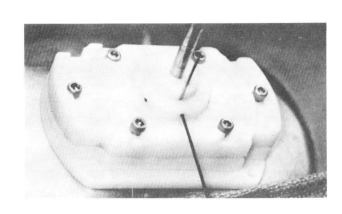
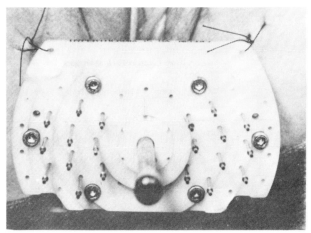

FIGURE 14-9

Nori–Hilaris–Anderson Template

This template is used at Memorial Hospital in advanced and/or recurrent carcinoma of the cervix (**Fig. 14-10**). It consists of a perineal template with removable parts, corresponding to its superior (urethral) and inferior (rectal) portions, and of a vaginal obturator, uterine tandem, and stainless-steel needles with stylets.

The insertion steps of this template are similar to the steps previously described for the Syed–Neblett template.

The assembled template-applicator without the uterine tandem and with the removable superior and inferior portions in place is shown in **Fig. 14-11.**

The assembled applicator-template with the uterine tandem, but without the superior and inferior parts, is shown in **Fig. 14-12.**

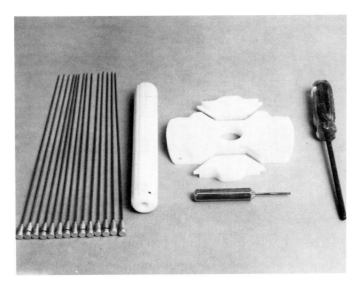

FIGURE 14-10

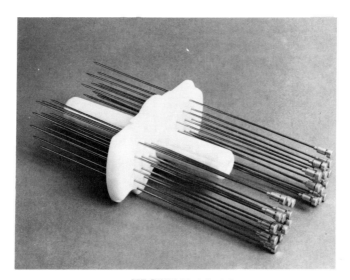

FIGURE 14-11

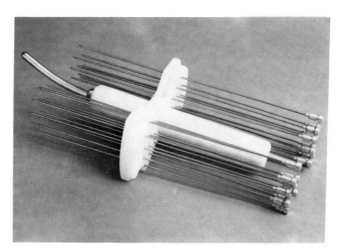

FIGURE 14-12

253

TREATMENT RESULTS

The ability to control local disease in cancer of the cervix diminishes as the tumor stage increases. It is, however, excellent in early stages. The Patterns of Care Study of the American College of Radiology underlined the association of recurrences with inadequate central doses, i.e., with failure to administer optimal intracavitary irradiation. On the other hand, the presence of complications was associated more with daily external beam doses than with the lateral and central doses used in brachytherapy.

The nineteenth volume of the *Annual Report on the Results of Treatment in Gynecological Cancer* sponsored by the International Federation of Gynecology and Obstetrics (FIGO) includes results of treatment on carcinoma of the cervix obtained in the 3-year period 1976 through 1978 in 120 institutions. The average survival by stage is 78 percent, 57 percent, 31 percent, and 8 percent (**Table 14-3**). The results, stage by stage, are better for the epidermoid carcinomas compared with the adenocarcinomas. Most of the deaths from cancer occurred within the first 3 years after treatment. During the period 1976 to 1978, 8804 patients with epidermoid cancer, not submitted to surgery, received intracavitary radiation. **Table 14-4** shows the 5-year results by conventional and afterloading methods. Patients treated by afterloading techniques seem to have better survival rates, possibly due to selection factors not clear in the report.

Perez et al. reported on a prospective randomized study in 118 patients with stage IB and IIA cancer of the cervix. All patients wre followed up for a minimum of 5 years or until death. Patients were randomly assigned to be treated with 1) irradiation alone or 2) irradiation (external pelvic and intracavitary) and surgery. The tumor-free actuarial 5-year survival for 40 patients with stage IB cancer treated with irradiation alone was 80 percent, and for 48 patients treated with preoperative radiation and surgery 82 percent ($p = 0.23$). The tumor-free actuarial 5-year survival in 16 patients with stage IIA cancer treated with irradiation alone was 56 percent and in 14 patients treated with irradiation and surgery 79 percent ($p = 0.13$).

TABLE 14-3

Stage	Patients Treated	5-Year Survival (%)
I	10,791	8430 (78)
II	11,599	6610 (57)
III	8,623	2671 (31)
IV	1,377	107 (8)
Total	32,428	17,483 (55)

TABLE 14-4

Intracavitary Method	Stage	Patients Treated	5-Year Survival (%)
conventional	I	1257	68.5
	II	2587	53.5
	III	2296	29.3
	IV	198	9.1
	Total	6338	46.3
afterloading	I	556	70.9
	II	1098	58.7
	III	742	41.0
	IV	70	17.1
	Total	2466	54.9

REFERENCES

1. Brown, S. G. Radiation therapy in the treatment of cancer of the cervix. In: Nori, D., and Hilaris, B. S. (eds.). *Radiation Therapy of Gynecological Cancer.* New York: Alan R. Liss, 1987, pp. 101–113.

2. Meredith, W. J. (ed.). *Radium Dosage, The Manchester System.* Edinburgh: Livingtone, 1967.

3. Henschke, U. K. Afterloading applicator for radiation therapy of carcinoma of the uterus. *Radiology* 74:834, 1960.

4. Henschke, U. K., Hilaris, B. S., and Mahan, G. D. Afterloading in interstitial and intracavitary radiation therapy. *Am J Roentgenol* 90:386–395, 1963.

5. Syed, A. M. N., Puthawala, A. A., Neblett, D., Disaia, P. J., Berman, M. L., Rettenmaier, M., Nalick, R., and McNamara, C. Transperineal interstitial-intracavitary "Syed-Neblett" applicator in the treatment of carcinoma of the uterine cervix. *Endocuriether Hyperthermia Oncol* 2:1–13, 1986.

6. Pettersson, F., Kolstad, P., Ludwig, H., and Ulfelder, H. (eds.). *Annual Report on the Results of Treatment in Gynecological Cancer.* Nineteenth Volume. Stockholm, Sweden: International Federation of Gynecology and Obstetrics, Radiumhemmet, S-104, 01 1985.

7. Perez, C. A., Camel, H. M., Kao, M. S., and Askin, F. Randomized study of preoperative radiation and surgery of irradiation alone in the treatment of stage IB and IIA carcinoma of the uterine cervix: preliminary analysis of failures and complications. *Cancer* 45:2759–2768, 1980.

8. Perez, C. A. Carcinoma of uterine cervix. In: Perez, C. A. and Brady, L. (eds.). Principles and Practice of Radiation Oncology, Philadelphia: J. B. Lippincott, 1987, pp. 919–965.

9. Fletcher, G. H. Cancer of the uterine cervix: Janeway lectures. *Am J Roentgenol* 61:225–242, 1971.

10. Fletcher, G. G. *Textbook of Radiotherapy, Third Edition* Philadelphia: Lea and Febiger, 1980.

CHAPTER 15

Brachytherapy in Cancer of the Corpus

CANCER OF THE UTERINE CORPUS

Cancer of the corpus tends to remain within the uterus for a long period of time, spreading by local extension initially within the endometrium. It may subsequently invade the myometrium and advance toward the endocervical canal. It can also spread paravaginally or paracervically, or it may extend directly through the myometrium to the serosa and to the peritoneal cavity. Because of the abundance of lymphatics as the serosa of the uterus is approached, deep penetration of the myometrium is usually associated with increasing incidence of lymph node metastasis. The lymphatic drainage of the upper part of the body of the uterus is along the course of infundibulopelvic ligament to the aortic, caval, lumbar, and the high common iliac lymph nodes. Once the lymphatic system in the cervical area has been involved, the spread of cancer mimics that of cancer of the uterine cervix. Lymphatic anastomosis between the body of the uterus and the round ligament are responsible for the rare metastases occurring in the inguinal area (**Fig. 15-1**).

Radiation therapy alone or in combination with surgery has been used successfully in the treatment of early cancer of the uterine corpus. The role of radiation therapy is determined largely by the stage of the disease when first diagnosed, by the degree of histological differentiation of the tumor, and by the size of the uterus. Preoperative external pelvic radiation is given in patients with an enlarged uterus, undifferentiated tumor, or spread of the disease to the endocervix. Preoperative intracavitary uterine radiation

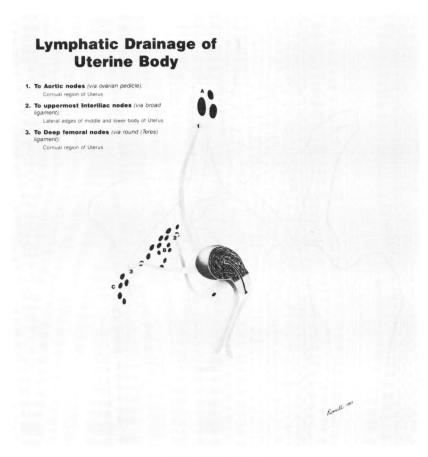

Lymphatic Drainage of Uterine Body

1. **To Aortic nodes** *(via ovarian pedicle)*:
   Cornual region of Uterus
2. **To uppermost Interiliac nodes** *(via broad ligament)*:
   Lateral edges of middle and lower body of Uterus
3. **To Deep femoral nodes** *(via round (Teres) ligament)*:
   Cornual region of Uterus

FIGURE 15-1

TABLE 15-1.   Cancer of the Corpus. Memorial Hospital Protocol for Operable Patients.

Stage (FIGO)	Preoperative* Irradiation	Postoperative Irradiation
1a G1 1b G1	None	a) Myometrial invasion ≲ ⅓: vaginal application (700 rads at 0.5 cm × 3 q 2 weeks)† b) Myometrial invasion >⅓: external pelvic (4000 rads/4 weeks) Vaginal application (700 rads at 0.5 cm × 3 q 2 weeks)
1a (G2, G3) 1b (G2, G3)	External pelvic (4000 rads/4 weeks)	Vaginal application (700 rads at 0.5 cm × 3 q 2 weeks)
II	External pelvic (4000 rads/4 weeks)	Vaginal application (700 rads at 0.5 cm × 3 q 2 weeks)
III	External pelvic (4000 rads/4 weeks)	Vaginal application (700 rads at 0.5 cm × 3 q 2 weeks)

*Additional boost doses with external are recommended if palpable nodal disease is found.
†Vaginal radiation is given utilizing the remote afterloading technique.

has become less popular because it failed to demonstrate improved survival or decreased pelvic recurrences; it is considered only for massively obese patients. Postoperative pelvic external beam and intracavitary vaginal radiation are given to patients who have not had preoperative radiation if the surgical specimen after hysterectomy shows that the tumor has penetrated the myometrium or has extended beyond it. Intracavitary uterine and vaginal radiation combined with external pelvic beam is given to all patients who are poor surgical risks or have extensive inoperable disease.

Vaginal radiation is an integral part of treatment management of corpus cancer. In most institutions, vaginal irradiation is given with vaginal colpostats designed to deliver between 4500 to 5000 cGy surface doses. At Memorial Hospital we have used the technique of high dose rate remote afterloading. The practical advantages associated with the use of this technique have been previously described (Chap. 3). Our treatment policy for the past 10 years is shown in **Table 15-1.**

Intracavitary Corpus Irradiation

This type of treatment will be illustrated using the Hilaris–Nori applicator. The applicator is inserted in the operating room under general anesthesia. The cervix is dilated up to a #18 Haynes dilator (**Fig. 15-2,** left); the cervix is grasped with a uterine tenaculum.

The applicator is inserted by the curved lateral tubes first, with one in each cornua (Fig. 15-2, right) followed by the straight central tube in between the lateral tubes (**Fig. 15-3,** left). If the central tube cannot be inserted, only the lateral tubes are used. The vaginal cylinder is linked with the uterine tubes by aligning the three uterine tubes with the central hole of the vaginal cylinder. The cylinder is pushed gently into the vagina until it reaches the uterine cervix. During the insertion of the vaginal cylinder, it is important to hold the protruding ends of the uterine tubes tightly to avoid their displacement and possible perforation of the uterus. The proper position and direction of the lateral tubes is checked by assuring that the end slit is oriented outwards (Fig. 15-3, right).

Packing of the vagina is not necessary but may be used if considered desirable. The labia majora are sutured with a silk mattress suture above the applicator; the suture is tied around the vaginal cylinder.

A tube is inserted into the rectum to allow subsequent localization radiographs and secured with tape on the perineum.

The radioactive sources are inserted into the applicator in the patient's room if manual afterloading is performed; for remote afterloading of the sources the patient is brought to a special suite.

The removal of the applicator, following the removal of the sources, is performed after the Foley catheter and the silk suture have been removed. The patient should always be examined for bleeding, lacerations, and so forth. The parts of the applicator are checked to make sure that each part has been removed.

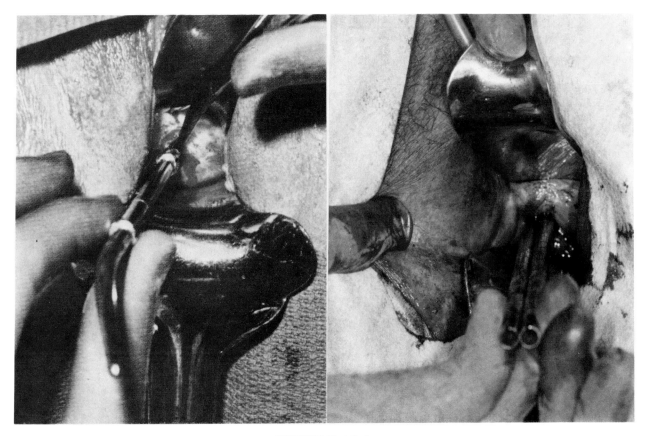

FIGURE 15-2

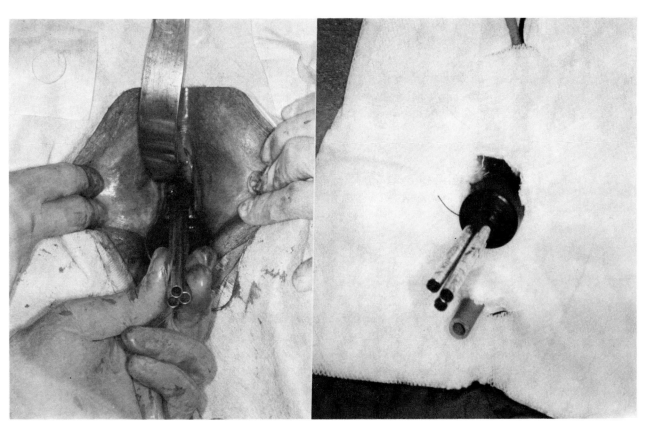

FIGURE 15-3

TREATMENT RESULTS

The nineteenth *Annual Report* includes the results of treatment from 1976 to 1978 in 13,581 patients reported from 94 institutions. The 5-year survival by stage is 75.1 percent for stage I, 57.8 percent for stage II, 30 percent for stage III, and 10.6 percent for stage IV (**Table 15-2**).

The 5-year survival was studied in 4518 patients with stage I carcinoma of the corpus, with respect to mode of treatment and grade of differentiation. The addition of postoperative intracavitary vaginal radiation has given better results in all histological grades than surgery alone or surgery and postoperative external pelvic radiation (**Table 15-3**). The authors of the *Annual Report* attribute these poorer results to the fact that external pelvic radiation was added only in patients with deep myometrial penetration who therefore had a worse prognosis.

The results of treatment in 300 patients seen in the Department of Radiation Oncology, Memorial Hospital, between 1969 and 1979 were reported in 1987. Multivariate analysis demonstrated that grade, stage, age, and extrauterine extension of the disease at the time of hysterectomy are the most important prognostic factors.

The 5- and 10-year disease-free survival in Stage IA is 96 percent and 91 percent, stage IB, 83 percent and 75 percent, and stage II, 77 percent and 71 percent respectively (**Fig. 15-4**).

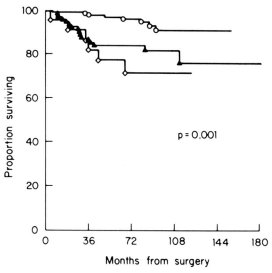

FIGURE 15-4

TABLE 15-2

Stage	Patients Treated	5-Year Survival (%)
I	10,285	75.1
II	1,885	57.8
III	844	30.0
IV	452	10.6

TABLE 15-3

Therapy	Grade I (%)	Grade II (%)	Grade III (%)	Grade Unknown (%)
Surgery alone	81.9	78.1	60.5	81.9
Surg & ICRT*	89.5	88.2	78.7	86.0
Surg & ERT+	76.9	73.2	55.7	77.9
Surg & both	83.4	75.9	60.5	78.9

*intracavitary vaginal radiation

+external pelvic radiation

REFERENCES

1. Pettersson, F., Kolstad, P., Ludwig, H., and Ulfelder, H. (eds.). *Annual Report on the Results of Treatment in Gynecological Cancer.* Nineteenth Volume. Stockholm, Sweden: International Federation of Gynecology and Obstetrics. Radiumhemmet, S-104 01 1985.

2. Shah, C., and Green, T. Evaluation of current management of endometrial carcinoma. *Obstet Gynecol* 39(4):500–508, 1972.

3. Graham, J. The value of preoperative or postoperative treatment by radium for carcinoma of the uterine body. *Surg Gynecol Obstet* 132:855–860, 1971.

4. Price, J., Hahn, G. A., Romingor, D. J. Vaginal involvement in endometrial carcinoma. *Am J Obstet Gynecol* 91:1060–1065, 1965.

5. Nori, D., Hilaris, B. S., Tome, M., Lewis, J. L., Jr., Birnbaum, S., and Fuks, Z. Combined surgery and radiation in endometrial carcinoma: an analysis of prognostic factors. *Int J Radiat Oncol Biol Phys* 13:489–497, 1987.

6. Brady, L. W., Lewis, G. C., Antonioades, J., Prasavinichai, D., and MacMurray, T. Evolution of radiotherapeutic techniques. *Gynecol Oncol* 2:314–323, 1974.

7. Graham, J. The value of preoperative or postoperative treatment by radium for carcinoma of the uterine body. *Surg Gynecol Obstet* 132:855–860, 1971.

8. Joslin, C. A. F., and Smith, C. W. Postoperative radiotherapy in the mangement of uterine corpus carcinoma. *Clin Radiol* 22:118–124, 1971.

9. Mandell, L. M., Nori, D., Anderson, L. L., and Hilaris, B. Postoperative vaginal radiation in endometrial cancer using a remote afterloading technique. *Int J Radiat Oncol Biol Phys* 11:473–478, 1985.

10. Perez, C. A., Knapp, R. C., Disaio, P. J., and Young, R. C. Gynecologic tumors. In: Devita, V. T., Hellman, S., and Rosenberg, S. A. (eds.). *Cancer: Principles and Practice of Oncology.* Philadelphia: J. B. Lippincott, 1983, pp. 1041–1055.

CHAPTER 16

Brachytherapy in Cancer of the Vagina

CANCER OF THE VAGINA

Most primary cancers of the vagina occur in women between the ages of 50 and 70 years. The most frequent site of origin is the upper vagina, but the disease may occur anywhere in the vagina and is often multicentric in origin. Secondary carcinoma of the vagina is very common, and such lesions usually arise from corpus carcinoma; they typically present just inside the introitus on the anterior wall immediately behind the urethra, and they may be due to retrograde lymphatic spread. Also, lesions may occur by direct invasion from cancer of the cervix, or there may be second-ary invasion by extensive cancer of the rectum or bladder. Very rarely ovarian cancer may erode through the pouch of Douglas.

Cancer of the vagina spreads primarily by direct extension laterally into the parametrial tissue and to the pelvic walls, anteriorly into the bladder, or posteriorly into the rectum; the main mode of spread is lymphatic (**Fig. 16-1**). The lymphatics from the upper portion of the vagina communicate with branches from the cervix and drain to the internal and external iliac lymph nodes. The lower half of the vagina drains to the pelvic and to the inguinal and femoral nodes. The anterior vaginal wall drains to the nodes on the lateral pelvic wall, especially the internal iliacs, and the posterior vaginal wall tends to drain to the deep pelvic lymph nodes, such as the inferior gluteal, the sacral, and the rectal nodes. Occasionally, metastases may be found in bones, lungs, and liver. Patients tend to die from locally uncontrolled disease leading to pressure on the ureters and to uremia, or more rarely from the effects of distant metastases in the liver or lungs.

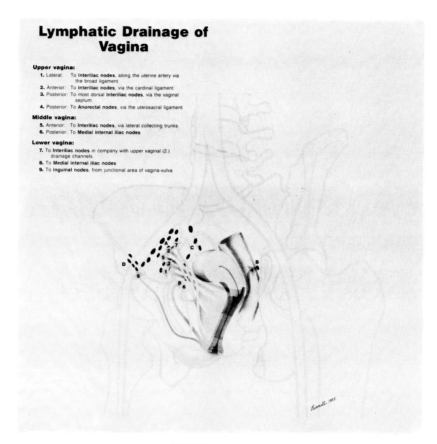

Lymphatic Drainage of Vagina

Upper vagina:

1. Lateral: To **Interiliac nodes**, along the uterine artery via the broad ligament
2. Anterior: To **Interiliac nodes**, via the cardinal ligament
3. Posterior: To most dorsal **Interiliac nodes**, via the vaginal septum
4. Posterior: To **Anorectal nodes**, via the uterosacral ligament

Middle vagina:

5. Anterior: To **Interiliac nodes**, via lateral collecting trunks
6. Posterior: To **Medial internal iliac nodes**

Lower vagina:

7. To **Interiliac nodes** in company with upper vaginal (2.) drainage channels
8. To **Medial internal iliac nodes**
9. To **Inguinal nodes**, from junctional area of vagina-vulva

FIGURE 16-1

Interstitial brachytherapy alone is adequate for the early lesions. When the lesion is large, more extensive, and/or poorly differentiated, external radiation should be considered. External pelvic radiation, especially in patients with bulky lesions, helps to sterilize the nodal metastasis and shrink the primary tumor to provide for an optimal brachytherapy application. Fractionated intracavitary vaginal boost treatments by remote afterloading can also be considered in place of interstitial brachytherapy. **Table 16-1** shows our current recommended therapeutic management for cancer of the vagina.

Interstitial Brachytherapy

The interstitial techniques applicable in this site are either the suture temporary technique using plastic catheters afterloaded with Ir-192 (**Fig. 16-2,** left) or the template technique using rigid needles afterloaded with either Ir-192 or Cs-137 (**Fig. 16-3,** left). Both of these techniques have been described previously (Chap. 3).

A single-plane or multiplane implant may be required. Implantation should be restricted to lesions involving no more than half the circumference of the vagina to avoid possible extensive necrosis. The uninvolved tissue should be kept away from the implanted region either by packing or by the use of an obturator. For lesions of the posterior vaginal wall, the rectal ampulla should be kept distended either with a 30-mL Foley catheter or a rectal obturator.

Target Dose. The target dose is calculated at a depth of 0.5 cm or the maximum tumor depth, whichever is larger, and at points in the rectum, bladder, and parametrium (Fig. 16-2, right and Fig. 16-3, right). CT-based dose calculations are to be recommended.

TABLE 16-1. Carcinoma of the Vagina: Memorial Hospital's Current Policy of Management

Stage	External Pelvic Irradiation	Interstitial Irradiation
I < 2 cm	None	6000–7000 rad in 6–7 days
I > 2 cm	4000 rad in 4 weeks	3000–4000 rad in 3–4 days*
II	5000 rad in 5 weeks	3000–4000 rad in 3–4 days†
III	5000 rad in 5 weeks + 1000 rad in 1 week boost	Implant to residual disease (2000 rad)
IV	6000 rad in 6 weeks	?Implant

*With complete resolution of the primary with external radiotherapy, can also consider remote afterloading fractionated intravaginal applications using Gamma Med II in place of interstitial therapy.

†Radiosensitizers either with the external radiotherapy or with the implant for extensive stage III and IV.

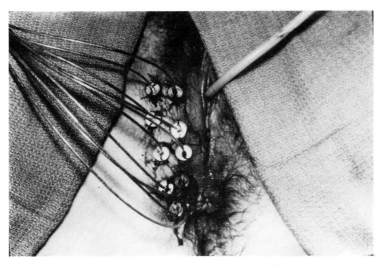
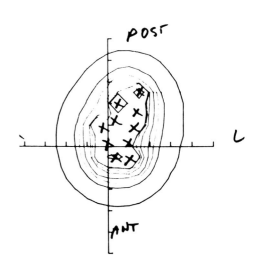

FIGURE 16-2

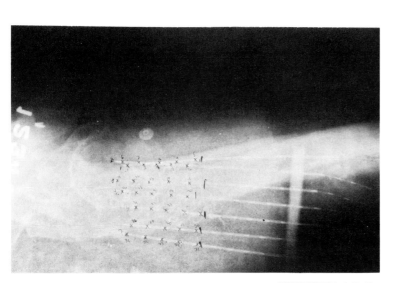
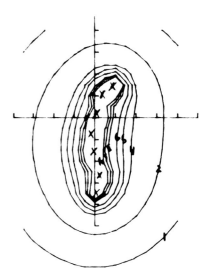

FIGURE 16-3

Intracavitary Brachytherapy

Intracavitary techniques with manual afterloading utilize a vaginal cylinder with or without a uterine tandem, loaded with Cs-137. For remote afterloaders, Ir-192, Cs-137, or Co-60 may be used.

It is important to select a vaginal applicator that provides good surface contact throughout the vagina for uniform dose distribution (**Fig. 16-4,** left). The patients are treated supine in lithotomy position to facilitate the placement of the applicator (Fig. 16-4, right). If a remote afterloading high dose rate technique is used, no sedation is required either before or during treatment, and all applications are performed on an outpatient basis.

Target Dose. The target dose is prescribed at a depth of 0.5 cm from the surface of the vagina or the maximum tumor depth, as in interstitial techniques. Orthogonal films are obtained to verify placement (**Fig. 16-5,** left); and isodose contours plotted at 4 to 5 dose levels permit dosimetric evaluation.

Figure 16-5 (right) compares the dose distribution of a treatment using a 6-cm high activity oscillating Co-60 source and conventional Ra-226 sources of the same active length of 6 cm—there is essentially no difference in dose distribution between these two treatments for the same total activity and time.

Figure 16-6 (left) shows the optimized dwell-time configuration of a remotely afterloaded Ir-192 source in a 2.6-cm diameter vaginal applicator. The treatment time generally depends on the diameter of the applicator and the length of the active sources.

Figure 16-6 (right) shows the vaginal mucosa in a patient treated with 700 cGy at 0.5 cm from the surface of the applicator every 2 weeks for a total of 3 applications (2100 cGy). Note the lack of any late reactions 5 years after treatment.

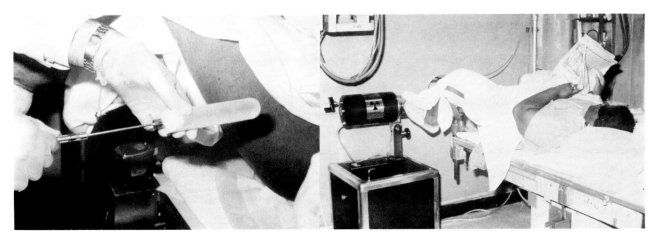

FIGURE 16-4

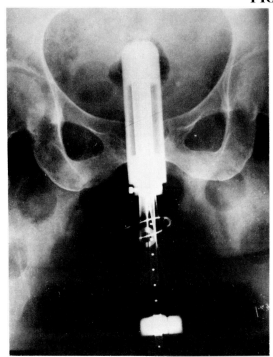

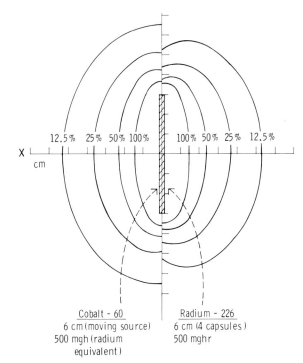

12.5%   25%   50%   100%   100%   50%   25%   12.5%

X
cm

Cobalt - 60   Radium - 226
6 cm(moving source)   6 cm (4 capsules)
500 mgh (radium   500 mghr
equivalent)

FIGURE 16-5

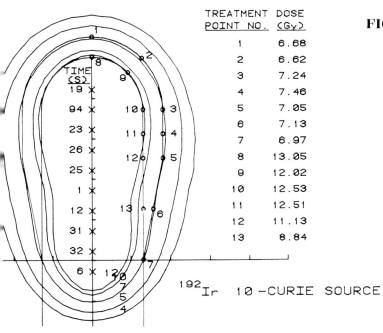

TREATMENT POINT NO.	DOSE (Gy)
1	6.68
2	6.62
3	7.24
4	7.46
5	7.05
6	7.13
7	6.97
8	13.05
9	12.02
10	12.53
11	12.51
12	11.13
13	8.84

^{192}Ir 10 −CURIE SOURCE

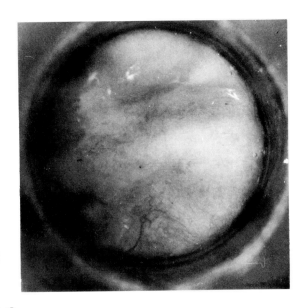

FIGURE 16-6

TREATMENT RESULTS

Table 16-2 shows the radiobiological equivalency of high dose rate radiation given by remote afterloading to conventional low dose rate radiation. If one accepts the validity of Orton's TDF concept, three vaginal applications of 700 cGy each, every 2 weeks, are equivalent to 3000 cGy given in 15 fractions of 200 cGy each.

The overall survival has improved from 10 percent in 1950 (Livingston) to 28 percent in 1968 (Frick et al.) to 45 percent in the most recent series reported by Perez, Brown, Prempree, and Nori (**Table 16-3**).

The value of brachytherapy alone or in combination with external beam radiation (for the more advanced stages) in achieving high local control rates is evident in the series of patients reported by Perez et al. Ninety-five percent of 38 stage I patients and 65 percent of 39 stage IIA patients were locally controlled.

The improvement in survival is generally attributed to 1) the advances and sophistication in radiotherapeutic techniques for external beam pelvic radiation, 2) the introduction of afterloading with computer planning and evaluation for intracavitary and interstitial brachytherapy, and 3) the development of new lower energy radionuclides as substitutes for radium.

TABLE 16-2. Remote After Loading Intravaginal Treatment Radiobiological Equivalent Dose

Oscillation Distance (cm)	Applicator Diameter (cm)	Dose Per Fraction (cGy)	Time-Dose Fractionation (TDF)	200 cGY 5 Times/Week Fractionation	Equivalent Dose (cGy)
5	3	500	29	200 × 9	1800
5	3	700	49	200 × 15	3000
5	3	800	60	200 × 20	4000
5	3	900	72	200 × 28	4800
5	3	1000	85	200 × 28	5600

TABLE 16-3.

Stage (FIGO)	Percentage Of:			
	Mallinckrodt Institute of Radiology 1953-1973 (114 pts)	M. D. Anderson Hospital 1948-1967 (76 pts)	University of Maryland 1957-1970 (71 pts)	Memorial Hospital 1949-1974 (36 pts)
I	81	69	83	71
II	41	68	64	66
III	30	27	27	33
IV	9	0	0	0
Overall	49	45	51	42

REFERENCES

1. Livingstone, R. G. *Primary Carcinoma of the Vagina*, McKelvey, J. L. (ed), Charles C. Thomas, Springfield, Ill., 1950.

2. Frick, H. C., Jacox, H. W., and Taylor, H. C. Primary carcinoma of the vagina. *Am J Obstet Gynecol* 101:695, 1968.

3. Perez, C. A., Aarneson, A. N., and Galakatos, A. Treatment of carcinoma of the vagina. *Cancer* 31:36–44, 1973.

4. Brown, G. R., Fletcher, G. H., and Rutledge, F. N. Irradiation of in situ and invasive squamous cell carcinomas of the vagina. *Cancer* 28:1278–1283, 1971.

5. Prempree, T., Viravathana, T., Slawson, R. G., Wizenberg, M. J., and Cucia, C. A. Radiation management of primary carcinoma of the vagina. *Cancer* 40:109–118, 1977.

6. Perez, C. A., Korba, A., and Sharma, S. Dosimetric considerations in irradiation of carcinoma of the vagina. *Int J Radiat Oncol Biol Phys* 2:639, 1977.

7. Nori, D., Hilaris, B. S., Stanimir, G., and Lewis, J. L., Jr. Radiation therapy of primary vaginal carcinoma. *Int J Radiat Oncol Biol Phys* 9:1471–1475, 1981.

8. Nori, D., Hilaris, B. S., Batata, M., Moorthy, C., Hopfan, S. Clinical applications of remote afterloaders. In: Hilaris, B. S., and Batata M. (eds.). *Brachytherapy Oncology*. New York: Memorial Sloan-Kettering Cancer Center, 1983, pp. 101–109.

9. Hintz, B. L., Kagan, A. R., Chan, P., Gilbert, H. A., Nussbaum, H., Rao, A. R., and Wollin, M. S. Radiation tolerance of the vaginal mucosa. *Int J Radiat Oncol Biol Phys* 6:711–716, 1980.

10. Sharma, S. C., Gerbi, B., and Madoc-Jones, H. Dose rates for brachytherapy applicators using ^{137}Cs sources. *Int J Radiat Oncol Biol Phys* 5:1893, 1979.

11. Perez, C. A., and Madoc-Jones, H. Carcinoma of the vagina. In: Perez, C. A., and Brady, L. W. (eds.). *Principles and Practice of Radiation Oncology*. Philadelphia: J. B. Lippincott, 1987, Chapter 53, pp. 1023–1035.

12. Harrison, L. B., Fogel, T. D., and Peschel, R. E. The treatment of primary vaginal cancer with combined external beam radiation and a simple, flexible intracavitary brachytherapy system (abstr.). *Endocuriether Hyperthermia Oncol* 2:219, 1986.

13. Syed, A. M. N., Puthawala, A., DiSaia, P., Berman, M., and Nalick, R. Interstitial intracavitary irradiation in carcinoma of the vagina (abstr.). *Endocuriether Hyperthermia Oncol* 2:219, 1986.

CHAPTER 17

Brachytherapy in Cancer of the Vulva

CANCER OF THE VULVA

The most common site of origin for cancer of the vulva is the medial side of the labium majorum. It is spread by direct invasion, first of the entire vulva and urethra, and then the perineum and anal margin in more advanced stages. A primary lesion of the clitoris is very rare. Vulvar lesions are more likely to be ulcerative than exophytic and indurated masses develop as a result of infiltrative and infective processes. The majority of vulvar cancers are squamous in type.

The main spread is lymphatic and large masses, exceeding the primary lesion in size by far, may develop in the inguinal regions. These nodes may infiltrate the skin and ulcerate with invasion of femoral vessels. Deep femoral venous thrombosis is a common complication. Posterior lesions of the vulva drain into a superficial inguinal nodal group along the inguinal ligament, into superficial femoral lymph nodes in the femoral triangle around the saphenous vein, and into deep femoral nodes along vessels under the inguinal ligament at the upper end of the femoral canal. The latter is referred to as the node of Cloquet or Rosenmuller. Anterior lesions of the vulva drain into the medial inguinal nodes. The lymphatics in the inner aspect of the labia minora drain toward the urethral orifice, follow the urethral lymphatics and join bladder lymphatics to drain into internal iliac nodes (**Fig. 17-1**). The vulva is a midline organ and lesions close to the clitoris, vestibule, or perineum may actually drain to lymph nodes on the opposite side. The overall incidence of positive lymph node metastases is about 40 percent.

The preferred treatment for carcinoma of the vulva is surgical resection. Radiation therapy is reserved for selected small lesions in older patients with complicating medical illness in technically unresectable lesions and in recurrent lesions. **Table 17-1** shows the suggested treatment plan, based on our experience, consisting of external pelvic irradiation and interstitial brachytherapy.

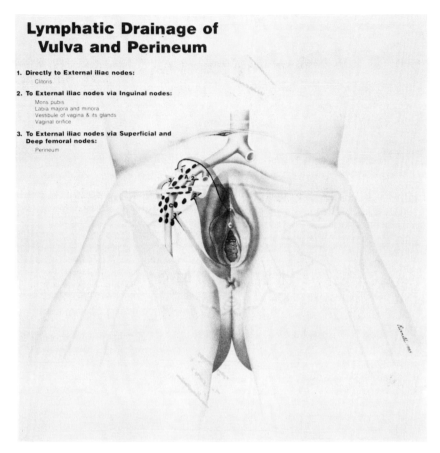

FIGURE 17-1

TABLE 17-1. Carcinoma of the Vulva. Memorial Hospital Suggested Radiation Therapy Treatment Plan

Stage (FIGO)	External Pelvic Irradiation	Interstitial Irradiation
I	4000–5000 rads to whole pelvis in 4–5 weeks	3000–4000 rads with removable implant
II	5000 rads to whole pelvis in 5–6 weeks	3000–4000 rads with removable implant
III	5000 rads to whole pelvis in 5–6 weeks plus boost to primary and bilateral groins with electrons; 1500–2000 rads in 2–3 weeks	Interstitial implant in place of boost therapy if bulky residual lesion present
IV	6000 rads to whole pelvis in 5–6 weeks. INDIVIDUALIZE	?Implant

Interstitial Brachytherapy

Because of the poor radiation tolerance of perineal and pelvic structures, external pelvic radiation is often combined with interstitial radiation procedures.

Vulvar implants are usually planar, consisting of a single or a two-plane arrangement. The percutaneous route is preferred in these implants, using either the basic temporary technique with plastic catheters or the template technique. In both techniques the implant is loaded with Ir-192 seeds in ribbons, although I-125 seeds can be substituted.

A temporary single-plane implant with plastic catheters in advanced vulvar carcinoma is shown in **Fig. 17.2.**

In interstitial implants, manually afterloaded with Ir-192 or I-125, the recommended dose rate in the central transverse plane is in the range of 40 to 80 cGy/hour (**Fig. 17-3**).

For remote afterloading techniques, intermediate or high dose rates with proper fractionation can be used.

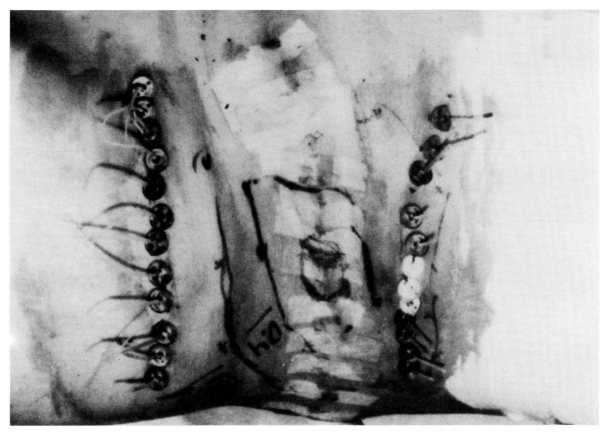

FIGURE 17-2

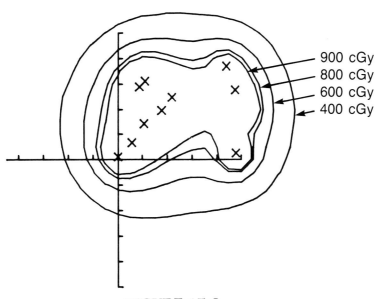

900 cGy
800 cGy
600 cGy
400 cGy

FIGURE 17-3

Temporary Ir-192 or I-125 implants using customized templates are preferred, whenever possible, in the management of large advanced lesions.

Figure 17-4 (left) shows an advanced vulvar lesion, recurrent after surgical resection.

Figure 17-4 (right) shows custom-made templates used to stabilize the rigid needles.

Figure 17-5 (left) shows the isodose distribution, displayed in the central transverse CT scan. The target dose rate (inner isodose contour), is equal to 2000 cGy/day. The x's correspond to the position of the needles.

Figure 17-5 (right) shows the same patient 1 year after treatment, without evidence of local disease. This patient died 1 year later of intraabdominal disease without evidence of local tumor.

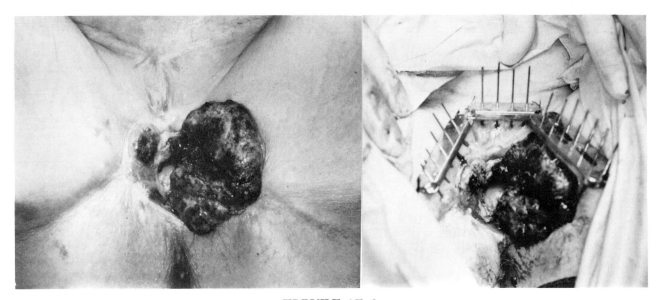

FIGURE 17-4

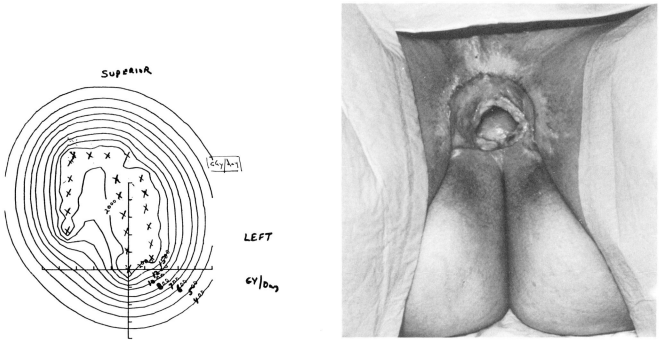

FIGURE 17-5

TREATMENT RESULTS

The nineteenth volume of the *Annual Report on the Results of Treatment in Carcinoma of the Uterus* reports on 2590 patients with cancer of the vulva. Surgery was the choice of treatment in early cancer of the vulva; radiation was given to patients with more advanced disease. The 5-year survival by stage was: 71 percent for stage I, 47 percent for stage II, 32 percent for stage III, and 11 percent for stage IV (**Table 17-2**).

Thirty-three patients with advanced primary or recurrent cancer of the vulva were treated at Memorial Sloan-Kettering Cancer Center from May 1950 to April 1979. The majority of these patients were treated by external radiation alone (23 patients); the remaining 10 patients were treated with either a combination of external beam and brachytherapy or brachytherapy alone. The external radiation dose ranged from 4000 cGy in 4 weeks to 6000 cGy in 6 to 7 weeks. When combined with interstitial brachytherapy, the external radiation dose was decreased to 5000 cGy, and was supplemented by a boost dose delivered by interstitial brachytherapy of 3000 to 4000 cGy.

The survival in group I (patients having recurrent vulvar cancer following surgical resection) ranged from 3 months to 11 years; two patients survived more than 5 years after radiation. The survival in group II (patients with stage III or IV advanced cancer of the vulva, previously untreated) ranged from 2 to 40 months; no patient survived for 5 years.

Results of treatment, utilizing brachytherapy for advanced vulvar cancer, reported by Tod, Ellis, and Helgason, range from 13 to 25 percent. More recently, Boronow reported a series of 33 patients, treated from 1968 to 1980, with a combination of surgery and radiation that included intracavitary brachytherapy. The actuarial 5-year survival with this approach was approximately 75 percent. The obvious advantage of this combination, according to the author, is the preservation of bladder and rectum associated with low morbidity and good local control.

TABLE 17-2

Stage	Patients Seen	5-Year Survival	Percent
I	781	558	72
II	733	346	47
III	844	270	32
IV	219	23	11
Total	2590	1198	46

REFERENCES

1. Plentle, A. A., and Friedman, E. A. *Lymphatic System of the Female Genitalia. A Morphologic Basis of Oncologic Diagnosis and Therapy.* Philadelphia: Saunders, 1971, pp. 15–30.

2. Pettersson, F., Kolstad, P., Ludwig, H., and Ulfelder, H. (eds.). *Annual Report on the Results of Treatment in Gynecological Cancer.* Nineteenth Volume. Stockholm, Sweden: International Federation of Gynecology and Obstetrics. 1985, Radiumhemmet, S-104 01.

3. Nori, D., Cain, J., Hilaris, B., Jones, W. B., and Lewis, J. L. Metronidazole as a radiosensitizer and high dose radiation in advanced vulvo-vaginal malignancies, a pilot study *Gynecol Oncol* 16:117–128, 1983.

4. Nori, D. Principles of radiotherapy in the treatment of cancer of the vulva. Nori, D., and Hilaris, B. S. (eds.). In: *Radiation Therapy of Gynecological Cancer.* New York: Alan R. Liss, 1987, pp. 191–198.

5. Ellis, F. Cancer of the vulva treated by radiation. *Br J Radiol* 22:513, 1949.

6. Tod, M. C. Radium implantation treatment of carcinoma vulva. *Br J Radiol* 22:508, 1949.

7. Helgason, N. M., Hass, A. C., and Latourette, H. B. Radiation therapy in carcinoma of the vulva. *Cancer* 30:997, 1972.

8. Boronow, R. C. Combined therapy as an alternative to exenteration for locally advanced vulvo-vaginal cancer: rationale and results. *Cancer* 49:1085–1091, 1982.

9. Pelepich, M. V. Carcinoma of the vulva. In: Perez, C. A. and Brady, L. W. (eds.). *Principles and Practice of Radiation Oncology.* Philadelphia: J. B. Lippincott, 1987, Chap. 54, pp. 1036–1043.

10. Miyazawa, K., Nori, D., Hilaris, B. S., and Lewis, Jr., J. L. Role of Radiation Therapy in the Treatment of Advanced Vulvar Carcinoma. *J Reproductive Med,* 28:539–541, Aug. 1983.

CHAPTER 18

Brachytherapy in Cancer of the Female Urethra

CANCER OF THE FEMALE URETHRA

Primary carcinoma of the urethra is rare, while urethral involvement by primary cancers of the adjoining organs is rather common. Carcinoma of the female urethra is usually a squamous cell tumor, although it can occasionally be a transitional cell type. Adenocarcinoma occurs rarely, and it arises from the paraurethral ducts and glands. Infiltrating tumors usually demonstrate early periurethral, anterior vaginal wall, and bladder base involvement.

Accurate assessment of tumor extent requires thorough clinical evaluation, including careful examination of the urethra, labia, vagina, and inguinal areas, cystourethroscopy, bimanual examination under anesthesia to evaluate extent of induration and fixation of the primary tumor, and to determine pelvic and inguinal lymph node status, and imaging studies, such as CT scans.

The radiotherapeutic treatment approaches include external beam radiation and intracavitary and/or interstitial brachytherapy.

The low incidence of lymph node and distant metastases in localized well differentiated lesions makes a high cure rate possible, if the primary site is adequately treated.

In a previous publication we have classified as *anterior* tumors located in the distal third of the urethra, or *entire* when more than the anterior portion of the urethra was involved (**Fig. 18-1**).

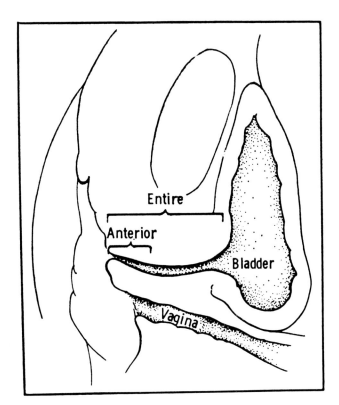

FIGURE 18-1

Brachytherapy Technique

A special urethral applicator, used by the authors for more than 20 years, has been described in Chap. 2. This applicator combines an interstitial implant around the urethra with an intracavitary application in the urethra and bladder (**Fig. 18-2**, left). The insertion of the applicator is done in the operating room under general anesthesia. The applicator consists of two acrylic plastic templates of the same diameter, six 17-gauge stainless-steel needles placed in a circular design around the urethra, and a central urethral stainless-steel tube. The needles are spaced 1 cm from each other and also 1 cm from the center of the template.

The patient is placed in the lithotomy position. A Foley catheter, with a stainless-steel tube inserted into it for stabilization, is passed through the central hole of both templates and is introduced into the bladder. The Foley bag is filled with 30 mL of radiopaque solution and is pulled back against the bladder neck. The proximal template is advanced against the urethral meatus and is fixed in this position by a thumb screw. The second template is positioned 2 to 3 cm from the first, to stabilize the needles. Next the six stainless-steel needles with sealed tips are inserted around the urethra through the peripheral holes of both templates.

The afterloading with Ir-192 seeds in ribbons is carried out following localization radiographs that ensure proper positioning of the applicator and computer isodose contours to permit dosimetric evaluation (Fig. 18-2, right).

At the end of irradiation the Foley catheter is deflated, the sources are removed first. The remainder of the applicator (needles and templates) is then removed.

Target Volume.   Includes the urethral lesion and a margin of at least 1 cm around it.

Target Dose.   The target dose is 6000 cGy in 5 to 7 days for tumors that are not larger than 4 cm, are of low histological grade, and are without regional or extraregional involvement.

For tumors that involve the proximal or entire urethra and measure more than 4 cm, and for tumors of high grade or with regional involvement, the whole pelvis, including the primary tumor and regional lymphatics, should be initially irradiated to a dose of 4500 to 5000 cGy. A boost dose of 3500 to 4000 cGy is given. Customized templates may be constructed (**Fig. 18-3,** left). CT-assisted computerized dose distribution is tailored to the tumor size and extent (Fig. 18-3, right). In this example the target dose (inner isodose contour) is normalized to 100 percent.

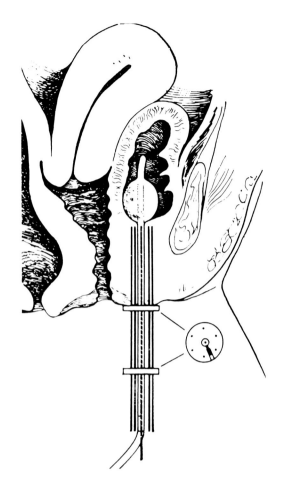
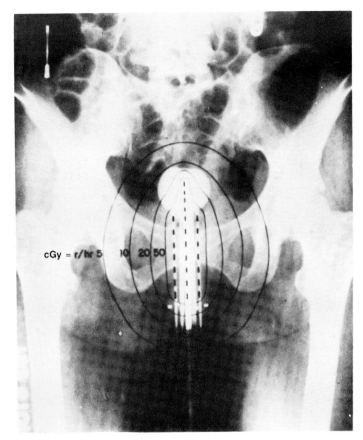

FIGURE 18-2

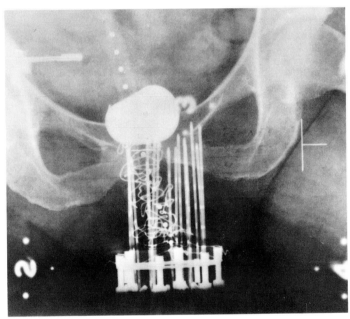
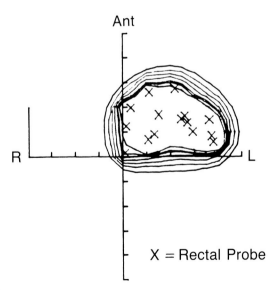

X = Rectal Probe

FIGURE 18-3

RESULTS

Table 18-1 shows the results of treatment in our 12 patients treated by the previous technique, according to primary site, tumor size, histological grade, and presence of involved regional nodes.

The 5-year survival rate without evidence of recurrence is 67 percent. Patients who have tumors located in the anterior urethra, which are smaller than 4 cm in size with low histological grade and without regional lymphadenopathy, have a 5-year disease-free survival ranging from 88 to 100 percent.

Declos et al. reported the results of radiation treatment in 38 patients, treated from 1948 to 1972, at M. D. Anderson Hospital and Tumor Institute. Fourteen patients (37 percent) were alive and free of disease at 5 years.

TABLE 18-1

Factors	Patients at Risk	5-Year Survival (%)
Primary Site		
anterior urethra	3	100
entire urethra	9	56
Tumor size		
<4 cm	5	100
>4 cm	7	43
Histological grade		
low	8	88
high	4	25
Inguinal nodes		
Uninvolved	9	89
Involved	3	0
TOTAL	12	67

REFERENCES

1. Grabstald, H., Hilaris, B., Henschke, U., and Whitmore, W. F. Cancer of the female urethra. *JAMA* 197:835–842, 1966.

2. Henschke, U. K., Hilaris, B. S., and Mahan, D. G. Afterloading in interstitial and intracavitary radiation therapy. *Am J Roentenol Radium Ther Nucl Med* 90:386–395, 1963.

3. Hilaris, B. S., and Batata, M. A. Cancer of the female urethra. In: Hilaris, B. S. (ed.). *Handbook of Interstitial Brachytherapy.* Acton, Mass: Publishing Sciences Group, 1975, pp. 235–239.

4. Batata, M. A., and Hilaris, B. S. Radiation therapy techniques in urologic cancer. In: Devine, C. J., and Stecker, J. F. (eds.). *Urology in Practice.* Boston: Little, Brown, 1978, pp. 785–792.

5. Nori, D., Hilaris, S., and Batata, M. A. Cancer of the urethra. In: Nori, D., and Hilaris, B. S. (eds.). *Radiation Therapy of Gynecological Cancer.* New York: Alan R. Liss, 1987, pp. 199–205.

6. Delclos, L., Wharton, J. T., Fletcher, G. H., and Rutledge, F. N. The role of brachytherapy in the treatment of primary carcinoma of the vagina and female urethra. In: Georege, F. W. III (ed.). *Modern Interstitial and Intracavitary Radiation Management.* New York: Masson, 1981, pp. 71–82.

CHAPTER 19

Brachytherapy in Pediatric Oncology

Cancer is the second cause of death in children younger than 14 years of age; solid tumors make up about half of these cancers (**Table 19-1**). Unquestionably in the last 20 years the outlook for these children has dramatically changed, mainly through earlier diagnosis and the institution of integrated multidisciplinary management resulting in impressive improvements in survival.

Reports from many pediatric cooperative groups, however, indicate disturbances in growth and development, and physiological impairment of organ function, following external beam irradiation, usually in conjunction with chemotherapy. Many of the reported complications are a direct result of large treatment volumes and high radiation doses, and they are inversely related to the age of the child.

Brachytherapy has not been used frequently in the management of pediatric solid tumors. On theoretical grounds, however, the integration of brachytherapy into the multidisciplinary management of pediatric cancers should be advantageous and it should minimize many of the adverse late effects observed with conventional external beam radiation.

The substitution of I-125 for Ir-192 temporary implants in our experience 1) permits significant reduction in radiation exposure levels to medical and paramedical personnel, 2) affords increased acceptance of the treatment by nursing staff and parents, 3) simplifies the nursing care of these children by the use of a lead apron that prevents exposure to protected areas (**Fig. 19-1**), and 4) decreases acute and, hopefully, late normal-tissue reactions.

Current indications for brachytherapy include selected solid tumors of the head and neck, gynecological and urological sites, and soft tissue sarcomas of the extremities. Brachytherapy is incorporated into therapeutic regimens that include chemotherapy, surgery, and moderate doses of external beam radiation.

TABLE 19-1. Pediatric Cancers

Cancer	Incidence (%)
Leukemia/Lymphoma	50
Brain	10
Bone	7
Neuroblastoma	8
Retinoblastoma	3
Rhabdomyosarcoma	5
Wilm's	5
Other	11

From J Ped Surgery 5:78, 1970.

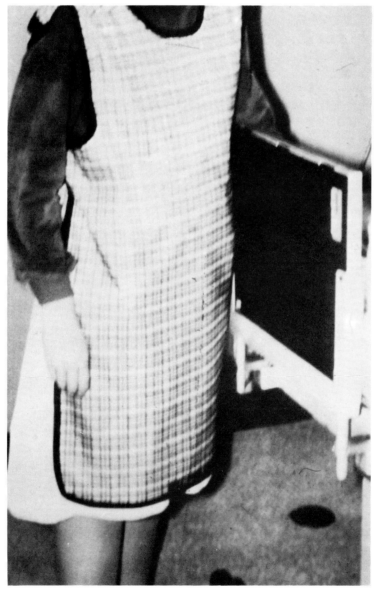

FIGURE 19-1

Temporary Interstitial Brachytherapy Technique

The preferred technique of interstitial brachytherapy is almost exclusively the temporary Ir-192 or I-125 basic or blind end technique. A permanent I-125 implant may be used occasionally for gross residual disease in deep-seated primary or recurrent lesions.

The procedure is usually performed under general anesthesia. Treatment planning is performed according to guidelines incorporated into New York system of dosimetry. The planar implant nomogram is used to achieve a peripheral dose rate of 1000 cGy/day.

Plastic afterloading catheters are positioned intraoperatively and secured at the skin, as described in Chap. 3. Localization films are taken with dummy sources to evaluate the target rate/day and the dose to critical normal tissues, i.e., skin, bone, and so on (**Fig. 19-2**).

Afterloading of radioactive sources is performed within 24 hours or 3 to 5 days later if surgery was carried out. Computer calculated dose distribution in multiple planes, perpendicular to afterloading catheters, can be superimposed to CT scans for more accurate dose evaluation and assessment (**Fig. 19-3**).

Room assignment is implemented to minimize radiation exposure not only to staff but also to other patients and visitors. Based on our experience for patients with temporary I-125 implants restrictions may be greatly relaxed. Standard lead aprons (0.25 mm lead equivalent) made available to both staff and visitors furnish essentially complete shielding of covered areas. In certain situations, shields of thin leaded material may be applied locally over the treated area to enhance protection further.

Restrictions regarding pregnant women and other children are strictly enforced.

Target Volume. Noninvasive imaging methods are used to determine the tumor extent. It includes the tumor volume and a margin of at least 1 cm around it. Potential pathways of tumor spread and tolerance of normal tissue are important considerations in outlining the target volume.

Target Dose. In temporary Ir-192 or I-125 implants the dose ranges from 4500 cGy in 3 to 5 days (tumor bed implant) to 6000 cGy in 6 to 7 days (implant alone). The target dose in permanent I-125 implants ranges from 12,000 to 16,000 cGy.

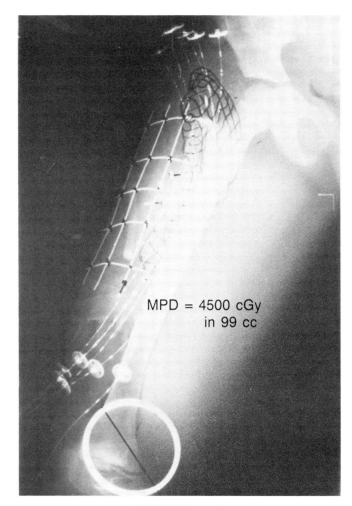

FIGURE 19-2

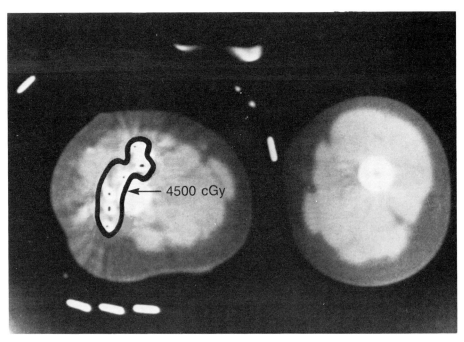

FIGURE 19-3

Intracavitary Brachytherapy Technique

The use of intracavitary brachytherapy in gynecological pediatric tumors allows the treatment of the entire length of the vaginal mucosa and paravaginal tissue while the remaining pelvic organs are relatively spared; the ovaries, in particular, receive a significantly lower dose. The treatment is usually combined with chemotherapy and conservative surgery.

The patient is examined under anesthesia to determine the extent of disease and to measure the length and diameter of the vagina.

A custom-made vaginal cylinder is prepared (**Fig. 19-4,** left). Localization orthogonal radiographs are taken (Fig. 19-4, right). Computerized dose evaluation is performed (**Fig. 19-5,** left). Remote afterloading with high-dose-rate Ir-192 is recommended because it permits the rapid administration of the treatment on an outpatient basis at a considerable psychological and financial benefit to the young patient and the family.

A 3-D target-isodose contour is recommended to facilitate the dose evaluation and determine if all the area at risk is included within the target volume (Fig. 19-5, right).

A target dose of 3000 cGy is prescribed at 0.5 cm from the surface of the applicator in 10 fractions.

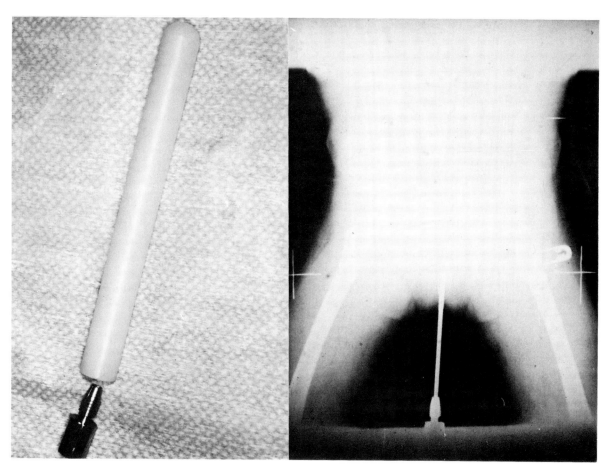

FIGURE 19-4

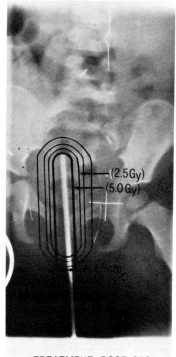

TREATMENT DOSE 25Gy

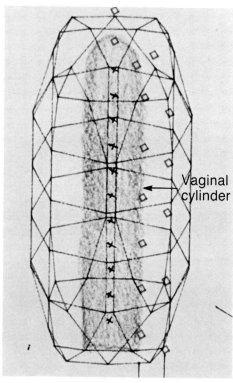

Vaginal cylinder

FIGURE 19-5

RESULTS

The Institute Gustave Roussy experience represents one of the largest reported brachytherapy experiences in the management of pediatric solid tumors. In 1985 Gerbaulet et al. reviewed the results of treatment of 45 children with malignant head and neck or pelvic tumors that were treated with Ir-192 temporary implants, chemotherapy, and, in some instances, partial resection and external beam radiation.

Twenty-three children had gynecological malignancies, 14 had head and neck tumors, 4 had urinary tract tumors, 2 had perineal tumors, and 2 had extremity tumors (**Table 19-2**). The long-term-year survival without evidence of disease was 78 percent (35/45 patients).

The late complication rate studied in 33 patients with a minimum follow up of 3 years, was 18 percent. These complications were related to either a high brachytherapy dose (7000 to 7500 cGy) or to a large target volume.

TABLE 19-2.   Institute Gustave Roussy Experience

Site	Patients at Risk	Patients Alive	Range of Survival (Years)
H+N	14	11 (79%)	2–8.5
GYN	23	19 (83%)	3–9.5
GU	4	2 (50%)	3–5.5
Perineum	2	2 (100%)	3–5.5
Extremity	2	1 (50%)	8.5
Total	45	35 (78%)	2–9.5

From Gerbaulet et al., 1985.

REFERENCES

1. Genest, P., Hilaris, B. S., Nori, D., Batata, M., Vikram, B., Hopfan, S., St. Germain, J., Anderson, L. L., Kim, J. H., and Alfieri, A. Iodine-15 as a substitute for iridium-192 in temporary interstitial implants. *Endocuriether Hyperthermia Oncol* 1:223–228, 1985.

2. Flamant, P., Chassagne, D., Cosset, J. M., Gerbaulet, A., and Lemerle, J. Embryonal rhabdomyosarcoma of the vagina in children: conservative treatment with curietherapy and chemotherapy. *Eur J Cancer* 15:427–532, 1979.

3. Martinez, A., Goffinet, D., Donaldson, S., and Palos, B. The use of interstitial therapy in pediatric malignancies. In: Vaeth, J. (ed.). *Frontiers of Radiation Therapy Oncology*. Vol. 12. Basel, Switzerland: Karger, 1978, pp. 91–100.

4. Knight, P. J., Doornbos, J. F., Rosen, D., Lin, J. J., and Farha, G. J. The use of interstitial radiation therapy in the treatment of persistent localized and unresectable cancer in children. *Cancer* 57:951–954, 1986.

5. Gerbaulet, A., Panis, X., Flamant, F., and Chassagne, D. Iridium afterloading curietherapy in the treatment of pediatric malignancies. *Cancer* 56: 1274–1279, 1985.

6. Fryer, C. J. H. Advances in pediatric radiotherapy in the last ten years and future proposals. *Cancer* 58: 554–560, 1986.

7. Horowitz, M. E., Pratt, C. B., Webber, B. L., Hustu, H. O., Etcubanas, E., Miliauskas, J., Rao, B. N., Fleming, I.D., Kumar, A. P., and Green, A. A. Therapy for childhood soft tissue sarcomas other than rhabdomyosarcoma. A review of 62 cases treated at a single institution. *J Clin Oncol* 4:559–564, 1986.

8. Nori, D., Hilaris, B. S., Kim, H. S., Clark, D. G., Kim, W. S., Jones, W. B., and Lewis, Jr., J. L. Interstitial irradiation in recurrent gynecological cancer. *Int J Radiat Oncol Biol Phys* 7:1513–1517, 1981.

9. Arbeit, J. M., Hilaris, B. S., and Brennan, M. F. Wound complications in the multimodality treatment of extremity and superficial truncal sarcomas. *J Clin Oncol* 5 (3):480–488, 1987.

CHAPTER 20

Brachytherapy of Ocular Melanoma

With the Collaboration of Sou-Tang Chiu-Tsau, Ph.D.

Ocular melanoma is the most common primary tumor of the eye, accounting for about 70 percent of all eye malignancies. It is located mainly within the globe, i.e., the choroid (75 percent), iris (12 percent), and ciliary body (10 percent). The overall incidence of ocular melanoma is similar in both sexes, showing almost identical age patterns. It is mainly a tumor of adults who have an average age of 50 years. Intraocular melanomas are not related to sun exposure. Studies have suggested a relationship between the cell type (spindle, epithelioid, or mixed) and prognosis—the spindle type having a better prognosis. Other studies indicate that size of the primary tumor is an important parameter with regard to prognosis. Distant metastases may involve any organ, although the liver is most common.

Ophthalmoscopic examination remains the most valuable diagnostic test in confirming the clinical diagnosis, especially in choroidal melanoma (**Fig. 20-1**). The diagnosis, in addition, is made by ancillary tests, i.e., ultrasound (**Fig. 20-2**), CT scan, and occasionally fluorescein angiography. According to Reese, iris melanomas rarely metastasize and can therefore be treated conservatively or by local excision. Choroidal or ciliary body melanomas, however, have at least 10 times greater mortality and therefore have been treated more aggressively by enucleation. In the last decade a better understanding of the natural behavior of these tumors, especially as related to tumor size, and the introduction of newer methods of treatment (i.e., high energy proton or helium particles) have encouraged local treatment.

Brachytherapy using ophthalmic applicators was introduced in the treatment of choroidal melanoma in an attempt to avoid enucleation and

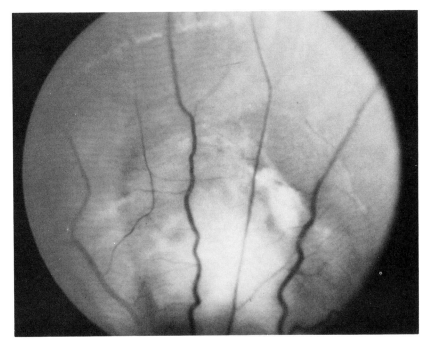

FIGURE 20-1

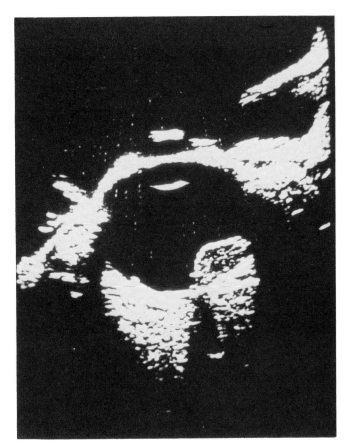

FIGURE 20-2

preserve vision. Stallard's results in the early 1960s suggested that survival following treatment by Co-60 ophthalmic plaques was similar to the survival obtained by surgery. More recently Co-60 plaques have been replaced by I-125 plaques because of the ease of protection of the noninvolved portion of the eye.

Brachytherapy with I-125 plaques is recommended for the treatment of solitary medium-sized tumors (less than 15 mm in diameter), tumors in the patient's only functional eye, and in patients refusing enucleation. Treatment of tumors larger than 15 mm, however, carries a high risk of scleral perforation and/or damage of the optic nerve.

TREATMENT PLANNING AND OPHTHALMIC PLAQUE DESIGN

Plaques used for the construction of ophthalmic applicators are either custom made or commercially provided. They are constructed of a gold outer plaque and a flexible plastic inner plaque. The Mayo Clinic eye plaque, one of the most common, is available in five standard sizes varying from 12 mm to 20 mm. Schematic drawings of a top view as well as a side view of the middle-size plaque (16 mm) are shown in **Fig. 20-3** (left).

Based on the actual I-125 seed strength, the distribution, orientation, and distance of the seeds from the surface of the applicator is determined. The seeds are assembled on the selected plastic inner plaque, which is then attached to the outer gold plaque. The completed plaque consisting of the plastic insert and the gold leaf is shown in Fig. 20-3 (right). The assembled plaque is gas sterilized prior to the application.

The number of I-125 seeds, their geometrical distribution within the eye plaque, and the activity of the individual seeds are determined by computerized optimization methods. Computed isodose contours, perpendicular to the plaque, are generated and plotted at various distances from the plaque. A typical example, for a 16-mm diameter plaque, is shown in **Fig. 20-4** (left). The corresponding radioautograph (Fig. 20-4, right) illustrates the well-localized irradiation around the I-125 plaque.

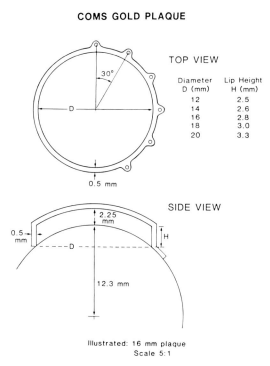

COMS GOLD PLAQUE

TOP VIEW

30°

D

0.5 mm

Diameter D (mm)	Lip Height H (mm)
12	2.5
14	2.6
16	2.8
18	3.0
20	3.3

SIDE VIEW

2.25 mm

0.5 mm

D

H

12.3 mm

Illustrated: 16 mm plaque
Scale 5:1

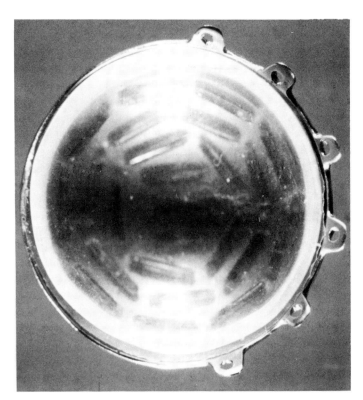

FIGURE 20-3

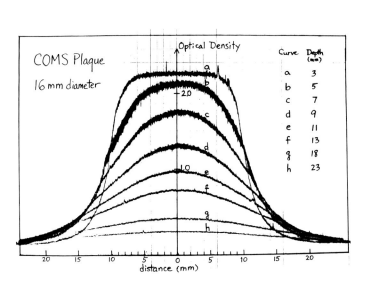

COMS Plaque

16 mm diameter

Optical Density

2.0

1.0

20   15   10   5   0   5   10   15   20
distance (mm)

Curve	Depth (mm)
a	3
b	5
c	7
d	9
e	11
f	13
g	18
h	23

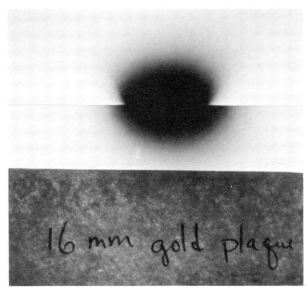

16 mm gold plaque

FIGURE 20-4

Ophthalmic Plaque Insertion

The insertion of the plaque is performed under general anesthesia. A small incision is made around the cornea over the tumor. The tumor is visualized by translumination through the lens and it is outlined on the sclera by cautery. The preloaded plaque is sutured, using the holes at the periphery of the plaque, over the tumor location marked previously by the cautery.

Target Volume. Includes the tumor base (diameter) and a margin of 2 to 4 mm around it. The tumor height corresponds to the thickness of the tumor (distance from the interior surface of the sclera to the apex of the tumor) and the thickness of the sclera (average 1 mm).

Target Dose. The target dose is 6000 to 8000 cGy calculated at the apex of the tumor. For tumors less than 5 mm in thickness, the prescription point is 5 mm from the interior surface of the sclera. To this distance, the thickness of the sclera should be added (i.e., 5 mm plus 1 mm = 6 mm). The dose rate at the prescription point may vary from 50 to 125 cGy/hour.

Dose to Critical Structures. The dose limiting structures are:

1. *Sclera*—dose is calculated in at least one point, usually at 1 mm from the central axis of the plaque.
2. *Optic nerve*—dose is calculated at the center of the optic disc. An effort is made to shield the optic nerve, whenever possible, by the lip of the plaque.
3. *Retina*—dose is calculated along a diameter of the globe passing through the apex of the tumor. It should not exceed 10,000 to 15,000 cGy.
4. *Lens*—dose is calculated at the center of the lens. Cataract can be expected with treatment of anterior tumors.

Computed dose distributions perpendicular to the plaque through the apex of the tumor are plotted. The tumor and normal structures are included to allow the determination of the target dose and the dose to normal structures (**Fig. 20-5**). The gold plaque effectively shields the I-125 radiation behind it, protecting the normal structures, as illustrated in the radioautograph shown in **Fig. 20-6**.

The patient returns, 3 to 5 days after the insertion of the plaque, to the operating room, and the plaque with the I-125 seeds is removed. Follow up is carried out at 6-month intervals, with fundoscopic examination, ultrasound, visual field examination, and acuity testing.

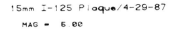

15mm I-125 Plaque/4-29-87

MAG = 5.00

Tumor Apex

Height 5.6 mm

Dose Rate 10 Gy/day
(42 cGy/hr)

Tumor Base

Dose Rate 42 Gy/day
(179 cGy/hr)

CODE	LEVEL
--	300.0 cGy/hr
--	200.0
--	100.0
--	80.0
--	60.0
--	50.0
--	40.0
--	20.0
--	10.0
--	5.0

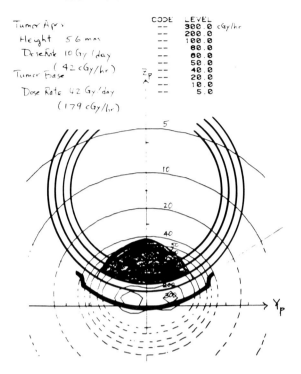

FIGURE 20-5

FIGURE 20-6

309

REFERENCES

1. Wilder, H. C., and Paul, E. Malignant melanoma of the choroid and ciliary body: a study of 2,533 cases. *Milit Surg* 109:370–378, 1951.

2. Norton, E. W. D., Smith, J. L., Curtin, V. T., et al. Fluorescein fundus photography: an aid in the differential diagnosis of posterior ocular lesions. *Trans Am Acad Ophthalmol Otolaryngol* 68:755–765, 1964.

3. Stallard, H. B. Radiotherapy for malignant melanoma of the choroid. *Br J Ophthamol* 50:147–155, 1966.

4. Zimmerman, L. E. Histologic considerations in the management of tumors of the iris and ciliary body. *An Inst Barraquer* 10:27–56, 1972.

5. Coleman, D. J., Abramson, D. H., Jack, R. L., et al. Ultrasonic diagnosis of tumors of the choroid. *Am J Ophthalmol* 91:344–354, 1974.

6. Reese, A. B. *Tumor of the Eye.* New York: Harper and Row Publishers, 1976.

7. McLean, I. W., Zimmerman, L. E., and Evans, R. M. Reappraisal of Calender's spindle A type of malignant melanoma of the choroid and ciliary body. *Am J Ophthalmol* 86:557–564, 1978.

8. Manschot, W. A., and von Peperzeel, H. A. Choroidal melanoma: enucleation or observation? A new approach. *Arch Ophthalmol* 98:71–77, 1980.

9. Migdal, C. Choroidal melanoma: the role of conservative therapy. *Trans Ophthalmol Soc UK* 103(1)54–58, 1983.

10. Chenery, S. G., Japp, B., and Fitzpatrick, P. J. Dosimetry of radioactive gold grains for the treatment of choroidal melanoma. *Br J Radiol* 56(666):415–420, 1983.

11. Korcok, M. Radiation, not enucleation for choroidal melanoma? *JAMA* 249(9):1123–1126, 1983.

12. Packer, S., Rotman, M., and Salanitro, P. Iodine 125 irradiation of choroidal melanoma. Clinical experience. *Ophthalmology* 91(12):1700–1708, 1984.

13. Weiss, J. S., and Albert, D. M. Intraocular melanoma. In: DeVita, V. T., Hellman, S., and Rosenberg, S. A. (eds.). *Cancer Principles and Practice of Oncology.* Philadelphia: J. B. Lippincott, 1985, 1423–1435.

14. Muller, R. P., Busse, H., Kroll, P., and Gast, E. Treatment of choroid melanoma with contact curietherapy using ruthenium 106. *J Fr Ophthalmol* 8(10):639–643, 1985.

15. Cleasby, G. W., and Kutzscher, B. M. Clinicopathologic report of successful cobalt 60 plaque therapy for choroidal melanoma. *Am J Ophthalmol* 100(6):828–830, 1985.

16. Gragoudas, M. Management of choroidal melanomas (review). *Int Ophthalmol Clin* 26(2):145–158, 1986.

CHAPTER 21

Interstitial Hyperthermia and Brachytherapy

With the Collaboration of Luis Linares, M.D.

Coley reported the antitumor effect of heat (hyperexia) in a communication published almost a century ago in the *American Journal of the Medical Sciences* (**Fig. 21-1**). Injection of the so-called *Coley toxin* is known to be an immunopotentiator with the side effect of high fever. An impressive illustration of its antitumor effects was included in the article and is reproduced here (**Fig. 21-2**).

It is only recently that we acquired a better understanding of the thermobiology of tumors and normal tissues. Concurrent technological advances in thermometry and in the design of hyperthermia equipment has made possible the clinical application of hyperthermia.

It is now well documented that temperatures higher than 41°C may have a lethal effect on cancer cells and that tumor cells, in general, are more sensitive to heat than normal cells. Normal tissues have a greater ability to dissipate heat by increased blood flow, while this mechanism is underdeveloped in many tumors, especially of large size.

The effects of ionizing radiation on tumors are enhanced by hyperthermia because of the presence of hypoxic cells, cells in S phase of mitotic cycle, and cells on low pH environment that are resistant to radiation but sensitive to heat. Hyperthermia may also interfere with repair of sublethal and potential lethal radiation induced damage.

Several techniques have been developed for the clinical application of hyperthermia. Systemic hyperthermia (whole body heating) is achieved by surface or extracorporeal heating. Regional hyperthermia is produced by either hyperthermic limb perfusion, water bath, microwave, or radiofrequency external application. Local hyperthermia can be achieved either by localized external application or by interstitial administration.

AMERICAN JOURNAL

OF THE MEDICAL SCIENCES.

SEPTEMBER, 1896.

THE THERAPEUTIC VALUE OF THE MIXED TOXINS OF THE STREPTOCOCCUS OF ERYSIPELAS AND BACILLUS PRODIGIOSUS IN THE TREATMENT OF INOPERABLE MALIGNANT TUMORS,

WITH A REPORT OF ONE HUNDRED AND SIXTY CASES.[1]

BY WILLIAM B. COLEY, M.D.,
ATTENDING SURGEON TO THE NEW YORK CANCER HOSPITAL; ASSISTANT SURGEON TO THE HOSPITAL FOR RUPTURED AND CRIPPLED.

FIGURE 21-1

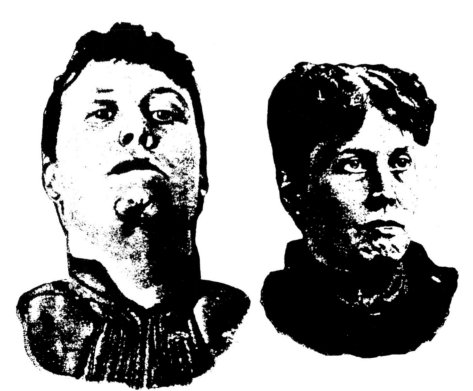

CASE VII.—Epithelioma of chin and floor of mouth. Before treatment.

Same patient one and a half years after treatment. Patient well two years.

FIGURE 21-2

Interstitial Hyperthermia Technique

The use of interstitial hyperthermia has attracted considerable attention since the early reports of Joseph et al. (1981), Manning et al. (1982), and Vora et al. (1982). The technique implies that the heating sources are implanted within the target volume.

The major advantages of interstitial hyperthermia over external hyperthermia are:

1. more uniform heat distribution within the target volume, especially in large tumors
2. more effective sparing of the neighboring normal tissue
3. only available method of heating deep-seated tumors

Interstitial hyperthermia can be combined either with conventional external radiation or low dose rate insterstitial brachytherapy.

Several systems are now available for interstitial hyperthermia, utilizing either radiofrequency- or microwave-induced heat (**Table 21-1**).

Hyperthermia Treatment Planning

The objective of treatment planning is to generate an optimal thermal distribution within the target volume. Computed tomography (CT scan) is taken at various levels to

1. outline the target volume, which includes the tumor volume and a variable margin around it
2. determine the number of electrode–needle pairs and thermocouples and their optimal distribution within the tumor and the neighboring normal tissue
3. select the sequence of application of the radiofrequency current to the array of stainless-steel pairs of needles

The target region is outlined on the CT scan or MRI if available (**Fig. 21-3**, left), as well as on the patient (Fig. 21-3, right).

Once the treatment plan is completed a full-scale model is developed, that contains the proposed number and position of electrode–needle pairs and thermocouples (**Fig. 21-4**, left).

The same information, as well as the sequence of heating of the pairs of needles, is provided in a schematic drawing to guide the brachytherapist during treatment (Fig. 21-4, right). This model is extremely helpful in better understanding the different temperature parameters within the tumor and normal tissue and their relationship to the different needle pairs at the time of heating.

TABLE 21-1. Interstitial Hyperthermia Systems

System	Frequency (MHz)	Thermal Conduction or Emittion	Thermometry
Radiofrequency	0.5–1	pair of rigid needles or plastic catheters	satisfactory
Ferromagnetic seeds	1.8	metal alloy seeds (i.e., Ni–Si)	not well developed
Microwave	300–900	coaxial antennae	satisfactory

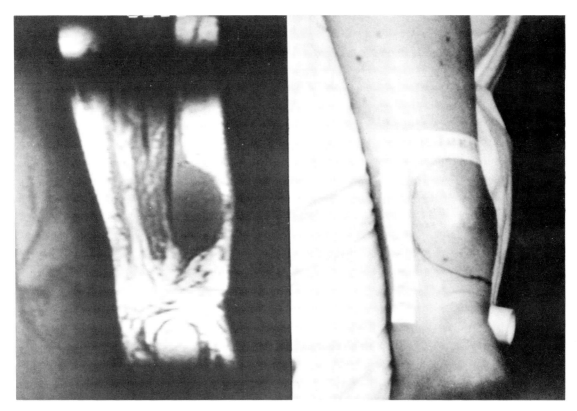

FIGURE 21-3

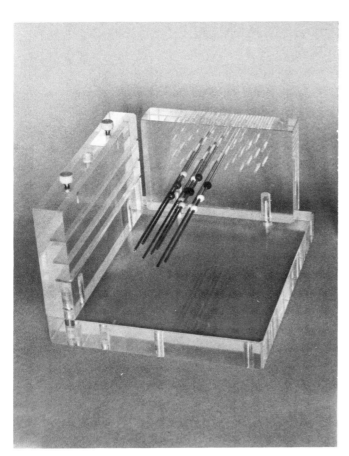

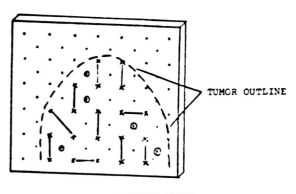

TEFLON TEMPLATE

TUMOR OUTLINE

X   X = ELECTRO NEEDLE PAIRS

X———X = SEQUENCE OF CONNECTIONS
        OF ELECTRO NEEDLE PAIRS

O   = THERMOCOUPLES OUTSIDE
       ELECTRONEEDLE PAIRS

FIGURE 21-4

Preparation of the Patient/Needle Insertion

The patient is usually treated under sedation with intermittent doses of Fentanyl and Diazepan, and an I.V. bolus of Ketamine for pain control at the time of insertion of the needles. The treatment area is prepared and draped in the usual sterile fashion.

The entry points of the stainless-steel needles (# 17 gauge) are marked on the skin. Two custom-made templates, made of acrylic plastic, are placed at the entry and exit points of the needles to help to guide the needles into the target area. Templates are used

1. to improve the accuracy of the needle insertion, and
2. to maintain the needles in parallel position and, therefore, improve the heat distribution during the treatment

The geometry of the electrode–needles, e.g., one-plane, two-plane, or volume arrangement (**Fig. 21-5**), is based upon the tumor size, location, and proximity of normal tissues.

At the completion of the insertion of the electrode–needles, a thermometry probe containing 2 to 3 thermocouples is introduced inside one of the needles of each needle-pair (**Fig. 21-6**, left). The remaining thermocouples are placed between the needle-pairs within the tumor and the surrounding normal tissue.

Once the thermocouples are in place, the electrode–needles are connected to the interstitial hyperthermia unit, according to the previously planned sequence (Fig. 21-6, right).

The selected temperature parameters are entered in the control panel: minimum 42°C and maximum 45°C, with a control sensor set at 43.5°C.

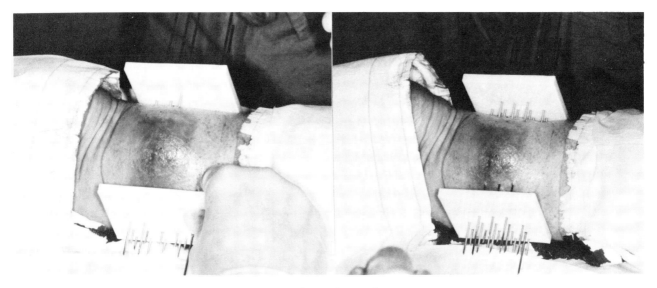

FIGURE 21-5

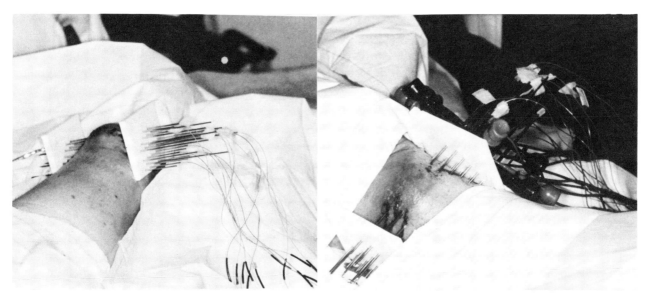

FIGURE 21-6

HYPERTHERMIA TREATMENT

The Radiofrequency Interstitial System used at Memorial Sloan Kettering Cancer Center (Oncotherm LCF 2016/2032) allows the selection of several treatment parameters in the following sequence (**Fig. 21-7**):

1. firing order of the electrode–needle pairs
2. dwell time assigned to each pair
3. percentage power level
4. temperature control sensor
5. temperature parameters: minimum, maximum, and control sensor's

Modification of any of the treatment parameters is possible during the heating session, including the percent power applied to the unit, the dwell time between needles, and the control sensor assignment to any of the available thermocouples.

Current temperature, monitored by each of 32 thermocouples, is displayed continuously on the hyperthermia unit's monitor before, during, and after the completion of the treatment (**Fig. 21-8**).

A cumulative temperature versus time plot of the control sensor(s) can be displayed, whenever needed (**Fig. 21-9**). It is thereby possible to monitor continuously the temperature during treatment and to adjust it to avoid hot or cold spots.

At the completion of the hyperthermia procedure the electrode–needles and the thermocouples are either removed and the patient receives external radiation, or the electrode–needles are replaced with plastic afterloading catheters that allow afterloading of radioactive sources for temporary insterstitial implantation.

RESULTS OF TREATMENT

Interstitial hyperthermia has been investigated in the last few years, in a variety of tumors, histological types, and anatomical sites. A review of the available literature, carried out by Emami et al. (1985), is summarized in **Table 21-2.** Analysis of these studies suggests that to maximize the local control

TABLE 21-2. Results of Interstitial Hyperthermia Treatment

Hyperthermia System	Patients at Risk	Complete Response	Complete and Partial Response
Radiofrequency	95	50%	79%
Microwave	82	62%	95%
Total	177	56%	87%

SEQUENCE PARAMETERS: File Name <u>CHAMP</u>

Firing Order	1	2	3	4	5	6	7	8	9	10	11	12	13	14	15	16	17	18	19	20
Needle Pair	<u>1</u>	<u>2</u>	<u>4</u>	_	_	_	_	_	_	_	_	_	_	_	_	_	_	_	_	_
% Dwell Time	<u>34</u>	<u>33</u>	<u>33</u>	_	_	_	_	_	_	_	_	_	_	_	_	_	_	_	_	_

Total Cycle Time <u>1</u>   Initial Power Level <u>3</u>

TEMPERATURE PARAMETERS: File Name <u>CHAMPION</u>

CONTROL SENSOR:
Number <u>12</u>   Temperature <u>43.5</u> deg C   Location <u>CENTER NEEDLE</u>

Treatment Duration <u>60</u>

Probe	A	A	A	B	B	B	C	C	C	D	D	E	E	F	B	N
Sensor	1	2	3	4	5	6	7	8	9	10	11	12	13	14	15	16
Location	T	T	T	T	T	T	T	T	T	T	T	T	T	P	S	
Maximum	45	45	45	45	45	45	45	45	45	45	45	45	45	45	45	42
Minimum	42	42	42	42	42	42	42	42	42	42	42	42	42	42	42	37

FIGURE 21-7

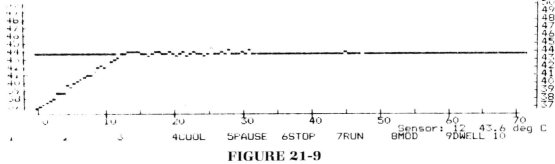

1   2   3   4COOL   5PAUSE   6STOP   7RUN   8MOD   9DWELL 10

```
STATUS - RUN                          SET TEMP.       - 43.5              CURRENT
RUN DURATION    77   min.             CONTROL HIGHEST - #  17   43.8      DATE/TIME
ELAPSED TIME   -  069:02              CONTROL LOWEST  - #  11   43.2      07/16/87
REMAINING TIME -  007:58              HIGHEST -        #  12   44.1       12:35:08
POWER LEVEL 100 %                     LOWEST -         #  24   27.6
```

1   2   3   4COOL   5PAUSE   6STOP   7RUN   8MOD   9DWELL 10

FIGURE 21-8

Sensor: 12 43.6 deg C

1   2   3   4COOL   5PAUSE   6STOP   7RUN   8MOD   9DWELL 10

FIGURE 21-9

1. the entire tumor volume must be included within the target volume
2. the minimum temperature within the target volume must be within the effective range of 42.5 to 43°C, and
3. a therapeutic radiation dose must be given beyond the heated target volume to effect subclinical disease that has not reached therapeutic temperatures

Although these early results are encouraging, further clinical studies are needed to determine the value of interstitial hyperthermia in combination with radiation therapy over radiation alone.

REFERENCES

1. Busch, W. Über den Einfluss welchen Heftigere Erysipelen Zuweilenauf Organisierte Neubildungen Ausüben. Verhandl Naturh Preuss. *Rhein Westphal* 23:28–30, 1866.

2. Coley, W. B. The treatment of malignant tumors by repeated innoculations of erysipelas with report of ten original cases. *Am J Med* 105:487–511, 1896.

3. Nauts, H. C. Pyropen therapy of cancer. A historical overview and current activities. In: *Proceedings of the International Symposium on Cancer Therapy by Hyperthermia and Radiation*. National Cancer Institute and Amer. Coll. Radiol. Univ. Maryland School Med. April 28–30, 1975, Washington, D.C., Chicago, ACR 1975, pp. 282–288.

4. Cavaliere, R., Ciocatto, E., Giovanella, B. C., Heidelberger, C., Johnson, R. O., Margottini, M., Mondovi, B., Moricca, G., and Rossi-Fanelli, A. Selective heat sensitivity of cancer cells. *Cancer* 20:1351–1381, 1967.

5. Leeper, D. B., and Henle, K. J. Hyperthermia: effects of different temperatures on normal and tumor cells. In: *Proceedings of the International Symposium on Cancer Therapy by Hyperthermia and Radiation*. Nat. Cancer Inst. and Amer. Coll. Radiology Univ. Maryland Schl. Med. April 28–30, 1975, Washington, D.C., Chicago, ACR 1975, pp. 282–288.

6. Leith, J. T., Miller, R. C., Gerner, E. W., and Boone, M. Hyperthermia potentiation—biologic aspects and applications to radiation therapy. *Cancer* 39:766–779, 1977.

7. Ben-Hur, E., Elkind, N., and Bronk, B. V. Thermally enhanced radioresponse to cultured chinese hamster cells. *Radiat Res* 58:38–51, 1974.

8. Hahn, E. W., Alfieri, A. A., and Kim, J. H. Increased cure rates using fractionated exposures of x-irradiation and hyperthermia in local treatment of ridgeway osteogenic sarcoma in mice. *Radiology* 113:119–202, 1974.

9. Robinson, J. E., Wizenberg, M. J., and McCready, W. A. Radiation and hyperthermal response of normal tissue in situ. *Radiology* 113:195–198, 1974.

10. Larkin, J. M. A clinical investigation of total body hyperthermia as cancer therapy. *Cancer Res* 29:2252–2254, June 1979.

11. Marmor, J. B., Pounds, D., Postic, T. B., and Hahn, G. M. Treatment of superficial human neoplasm by local hyperthermia induced by ultrasound. *Cancer* 43:188–197, 1979.

12. Kim, J. H., and Hahn, E. W. Clinical and biological studies of localized hyperthermia. *Cancer Res* 39:2258–2261, June 1979.

13. Mitsuyuki, A., Masahiro, H., and Masaji, T. Clinical experience with hyperthermia combined with radiation in treatment of cancer. *Cancer Treat Symp* 1:95–101, 1983.

14. Yatvin, M. Hyperthermia and local anesthetics: potentiation of survival of tumor bearing mice. *Science* 205:195–196, 1979.

15. Warren, S. Preliminary study of the effect of artificial fever upon hopeless tumor cases. *Am J Roentgenol* 33: 75–87, 1935.

16. Kare, K., and Hahn, G. M. Differential heat response of normal and transformed human cells in tissue culture. *Nature* 30:255–278, 1975.

17. Leveen, H. H., Wapnick, S., Piccone, V., Falk, G., and Ahmed, N. Tumor eradication by radiofrequency therapy. *JAMA* 235: 2198–2200, 1976.

18. Dewey, W. C., Hopweed, L. E., Sapareto, S. A., and Gerwick, L. E. Cellular responses to combinations of hyperthermia and radiation. *Radiology* 123:463–474, 1977.

19. Hahn, G. M. Potential for therapy of drugs and hyperthermia. *Cancer Res* 39:2264–2268, 1979.

20. Chen, T. T., and Heidelberg, C. Quantitative studies on the malignant transformation of mouse prostate cells by carcinogenic hydrocarbons in vitro. *Int J Cancer* 4:166–178, 1969.

21. Stehlin, J. S., Jr., Giovanella, B. C., De Ipoly, P. D., and Anderson, R. F. Results of eleven years' experience with heated perfusion for melanoma of the extremities. *Cancer Res* 39:2255–2257, June 1979.

22. Stehlin, J. S., Giovanella, B. C., De Ipoly, P. D., Muenz, L., and Anderson, B. A. Results of hyperthermic perfusion for melanoma of the extremities. *Surg. Gynecol Obstet* 140:338–348, 1975.

23. Kim, J. H. Combined hyperthermia and radiation therapy in cancer treatment: current status. *Cancer Invest* 2(1), 69–80, 1984.

24. Kim, J. H., Hahn, G. M., and Ahmed, S. Combination hyperthermia and radiation therapy for malignant melanoma. *Cancer* 50:478–482, 1982.

25. Emami, B., Marks, J. E., Perez, C. A., Nussbaum, G. H., Leybovich, L., and Von Gerichten, D. Interstitial thermoradiotherapy in the treatment of recurrent/residual malignant tumors. *Am J Clin Oncol* 7:699–704, 1984.

26. Surwit, E. A., Manning, M. R., Aristizabal, S. A., Oleson, J. R., and Cetas, T. C. Interstitial thermoradiotherapy in recurrent gynecologic malignancies. *Gynecol Oncol* 15:95–102, 1983.

27. Coughlin, C. T., Douple, E. B., Strohben, J. W., Eaton, N. L., Trembly, B. S., and Wong, T. Z. Interstitial hyperthermia in combination with brachytherapy. *Radiology* 148:285–288, 1983.

28. Cosset, J. M., Dutreix, J., Dufour, J., Janoray, P. Damia, E., Haie, C., and Clarke, D. Combined interstitial hyperthermia and brachytherapy: Institut Gustave Roussy technique and preliminary results. *Int J Radiat Oncol Biol Phys* 10:307–312, 1984.

29. Abe, M., Hiraoka, M., and Takahashi, M. Clinical experience with hyperthermia combined with radiation treatment of cancer. *Cancer Treat Symp* 1:95–101, 1983.

30. Vora, N., Forell, B., Joseph, C., Lipsett, J., and Archambeau, J. Interstitial implant with interstitial hyperthermia. *Cancer* 50:2518–2523, 1982.

31. Emami, B., Perez, C. A. Interstitial thermoradiotherapy—an overview. *Endocuriether Hyperthermia Oncol* 1(1):35–40, 1985.

Brachytherapy Terminology

1. *Absorbed Dose (symbol D):* The amount of energy imparted by ionizing radiation per unit mass of irradiated material at the point of interest. The SI unit of absorbed dose is the *gray* (symbol *Gy*). The concept of absorbed dose is very general and applies to any type of ionizing particles, charged and uncharged, and to any type of material.

2. *Absorbed Dose Rate (dD/dt):* The increment of absorbed dose in unit time interval, typically in centigrays/hour or grays/day.

3. *Activity (symbol A):* The number of nuclear transformations occurring in a given amount of a radioactive nuclide in unit time. The SI unit of activity is the *becquerel (Bq)*; a special unit is the *curie (Ci)*.

4. *Air–Kerma-Rate Constant (symbol Tδ):* The air–kerma-rate due to photons of energy greater than δ at unit distance from a point source of radioactive nuclide of units activity, typically in units of microgray square-meters/millicurie hours.

5. *Air–Kerma Strength (symbol S):* For specifying brachytherapy source strength, the product of air–kerma rate in free space and the square of distance from the source center along the transverse axis, at distances large enough that both source and detector can be treated as points. Recommended units are microgray meters-squared/hour.

6. *Attenuation:* The process by which radiation is reduced in intensity when passing through material. It is the combination of absorption and scattering processes.

7. *Average Dimension:* The average value of three mutually perpendicular measured dimensions of the target volume.

322

8. *Average or Mean Life (symbol T):* The length of time required for all of the atoms of a sample of a radioactive substance to decay if the rate were constant and equal to the initial rate of decay. Mathematically: $T = 1.44T_{1/2}$, also $T = 1/\lambda$.

9. *Becquerel (symbol Bq):* SI unit of activity: 1 Bq = 1/s, i.e., one decay event per second.

10. *Brachytherapy (therapy at short distances):* The treatment of disease with sealed radioactive sources placed near or inserted directly into the diseased region.

11. *Curie (symbol Ci):* Special unit of activity that continues in use while SI units are phased in. 1 Ci = $3 \cdot 7 \cdot 10^{10}$/s (exactly). Submultiples: (millicurie) 1mCi = $3 \cdot 7 \cdot 10^7$/s; (microcurie) 1 μCi = $3 \cdot 7 \cdot 10^4$/s.

12. *Decay Constant (symbol λ):* A characteristic constant for any radioactive substance, independent of any chemical and/or physical condition that is mathematically the fractional number of atoms of a radioactive sample decaying per unit time or the probability that a single atom will decay in unit time. $\lambda \cdot T = 1$; $\lambda T_{1/2} = 0.693$

13. *Excitation:* A process in which an atomic electron is raised to an outer unfilled shell.

14. *Exposure (symbol X):* The physical quantity expressing the ability of photons to ionize air. It serves as a measure of the output of radioactive sources. The SI unit of exposure is 1C/kg (1 coulomb per kilogram of air). The special unit of exposure, the *roentgen (R)*, may be used temporarily. The concept of exposure applies only to photons and only to one material—air.

15. *Exposure Rate (dX/dt):* The increment of exposure in unit time interval, typically in roentgens/hour.

16. *Exposure Rate Constant (symbol Tδ):* The product of exposure rate and the square of the distance from a point radionuclide source of unit activity. Both x-rays and gamma rays are included in the exposure rate.

17. *Gray (Gy):* The SI unit of absorbed dose and of kerma. 1Gy = 1J/kg (one joule/kilogram).

18. *Half Life $T_{1/2}$:* The time required for the decay of one half of the atoms of a sample of a radioactive substance. Also, the time required for a radioactive substance to lose 50 percent of its activity.

19. *Integral Dose:* Total radiation enery deposited in the irradiated material. Measured in gramrads or kilogram grays (same as 1 J).

20. *Ionization:* A process involving the liberation of one or more electrons from a parent atom or molecule.

21. *Ionizing Radiation:* Charged particles (negative or positive electrons, protons, or other heavy ions) and/or uncharged particles (photons, neutrons) energetic enough to cause ionization.

22. *Irradiated Volume:* The volume (larger than the treatment volume) that receives an absorbed dose that is considered significant in relation to tissue tolerance.

23. *Isodose Curve (or Surface):* A curve (or surface) depicting loci of identical radiation dose in an irradiated material.

24. *Kerma (symbol K):* Kerma derives from an acronym *KERM* for *kinetic energy released per unit mass* (the a has been added for pho-

netic reasons) and represents the sum of the initial kinetic energies of all the charged ionizing particles liberated by uncharged ionizing particles per unit mass of irradiated material at the point of interest. The SI unit of kerma is the gray. The concept of kerma applies to any material, but is restricted to uncharged ionizing particles (photons or neutrons). The concept of kerma is less obscure if one realizes that the transfer of energy from a photon beam, for example, to a medium takes place in two stages. In the first stage the photons interact with the atoms of the medium, liberating atomic electrons that are set in motion with certain initial kinetic energies. The second stage involves the transfer to the medium of the kinetic energy of the electrons through processes of ionization and excitation. Kerma involves only the first stage.

25. *Kerma Rate (dK/dt):* The increment of kerma in unit time interval, in gray/second or rads/second.

26. *Matched Peripheral Dose:* Dose for which the contour volume is equal to the volume of an ellipsoid with the same dimensions (along its axes) as the measured, mutually perpendicular dimensions of the target volume.

27. *Milligram-Radium Equivalent:* It has been common practice to specify the activity of brachytherapy sources in terms of equivalent mass of radium, where equivalence means the number of milligrams of radium (in a point source filtered by 0.5 mm platinum) that will produce the same exposure rate at a given distance as the source in question.

28. *Minimum Peripheral Dose:* The minimum dose on the surface of the target volume.

29. *Nuclide:* A species of atom with a specified number of neutrons and protons in its nucleus.

30. *Rad:* Special unit of absorbed dose and of kerma; superseded by the gray. 1 rad $= 100$ erg/g $= 10^{-2}$ Gy.

31. *Roentgen (R; r from 1928 to 1961):* Special unit of exposure that may be used temporarily. 1 R $= 2.58 \times 10^{-4}$ C/kg or 1 R $= 1$ esu of charge/ 0.001293 g of air $= 1$ esu/cm^3 air at STP.

32. *SI System of Units:* At the Eleventh General Conference on Weights and Measures convened in Paris during October 1960, the metric system of units (based on the meter, kilogram, second, ampere, kelvin, mole, and candela) was given the name *International System of Units* and the abbreviation *SI* in all languages.

33. *Target Dose:* The minimum dose planned for a target volume.

34. *Target Volume:* A contiguous region of tissue for which a prescribed minimum dose is planned. Also, the volume of this region. If a tumor volume has been defined, it will generally be enclosed completely by the target volume.

35. *Treatment Dose:* The minimum dose achieved within the target volume.

36. *Treatment Volume:* The region enclosed by the treatment isodose surface. Also, the volume of this region.

37. *Tumor Volume:* A region of tissue known to contain cancer and for which treatment is planned. Also, the volume of this region.

INDEX